Yoga Nidra Scripts 2

Praise for *Yoga Nidra Scripts 2*

"Compassionately written and a wonderful work of art... I had feelings of enlightenment even reading the words... So different to what I have experienced before."
 – Liz Burkitt, Yoga Teacher & Holistic Health Coach, EB Yoga & Health

"Love it. The cadence is poetic... it's simple to follow... reassuring language. It's the perfect tool. I've recommended the first *Yoga Nidra Scripts* book to the Moms of the youth I've been working with in my Reiki practice and will do the same with this book."
 – Jane MacPherson Bsc Kin., Reiki Master & founder of See Jane Heal

"An excellent second serving of Tamara's first book... a huge menu of delicious scripts for my yoga students who are hungry for relaxation and meditation. I love how each script is presented with complimentary pairings of asanas, pranayama, and mudras to satiate the appetite of the mind, body, and soul. This book will have your students returning for more helpings!"
 – Erin O'Neill, RYT 500, Erin O'Neill Yoga & Wellness

"A game changer... each script is thoughtfully written with a theme, structure, even well-placed pauses. You can guide your class effortlessly and safely from the physical body to the causal subtle body, one beautiful breath at a time. A must-have in my reference library. Teach a short class or an extended 45 minutes and feel confident that you and your clients will benefit either way."
 – Rosemarie Williams, RYT 500, Certified Aromatherapist, TanessaRose

"*Yoga Nidra Scripts 2* is a beautiful guide for yoga teachers, practitioners, and all types of healers. It will help guide and support you with inspiration, compassion, and self-care for all individuals... a must-have."
 – Amanda J. Carnes, RYT 500, Reiki Master Teacher, OM SHA Healings

Yoga Nidra Scripts 2

22 More Meditations for Effortless Relaxation, Rejuvenation and Reconnection

Tamara Verma
(Tamara Skyhawk)

For my beautiful community of yogis, friends and family. Thank you for being a constant source of inspiration and encouragement.

Disclaimer

This book is not intended to treat, heal or prescribe. The information contained herein is in no way to be considered as a substitute for a consultation with a duly licensed health care professional.

All Rights Reserved.

No part of this book may be reproduced in any form or by any electronic or mechanical means including information storage and retrieval systems without permission in writing from the publisher, except by a reviewer who may quote brief passages in a review.

Author: Tamara Verma *(Tamara Skyhawk)*

Copyright: © 2021 by Tamara Verma *(Tamara Skyhawk)*

Publisher: RTV Yoga Inc.

ISBN: 978-1-7774888-2-6 (paperback), 978-1-7774888-3-3 (e-book)

First Edition 2021

Contents

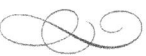

Author's Note VII

About This Book IX

Tips For Leading Yoga Nidra XI

Anytime Comfort *(15 Min.)* 1

Anytime Tension Release *(15 Min.)* 7

Anytime Soothing *(15 Min.)* 13

Anytime Warming *(15 Min.)* 19

Anytime Cooling *(15 Min.)* 26

Permission To Rest *(20 Min.)* 32

Inspire & Energize (Kapha Pacifying) *(20 Min.)* 39

Magical Morning *(20-25 Min.)* 46

Restful Night *(20-30 Min.)* 55

Courageous Confidence *(25 Min.)* 62

Fresh Start *(25 Min.)* 70

Pure Abundance *(25 Min.)* 80

Tranquility & Ease (Pitta Pacifying) *(25 Min.)* 88

Steadiness & Support (Vata Pacifying) *(25-30 Min.)* 96

Peaceful Orchard *(25-30 Min.)* 106

Vibrancy Rising *(25-35 Min.)* 114

The Getaway *(30 Min.)* 124

In The Loving Arms Of Mother Earth *(30-35 Min.)* 133

Sacred Pilgrimage *(30-40 Min.)* 144

Expanding Identity *(35-40 Min.)* 154

Summer Meadow *(35-45 Min.)* 164

Awakening Creativity *(35-55 Min.)* 177

Author's Note

Soon after the successful launch of my first book, *Yoga Nidra Scripts*, I started to receive requests for another book of Yoga Nidra scripts. And frankly, I wanted more scripts for my own teaching practice as well. So here we are – an abundance of new scripts, to use for the never-ending abundance of human feelings, situations and needs.

In creating this book, I wanted it to be a seamless continuation of the first, offering more scripts to help people effortlessly relax, rejuvenate and reconnect.

My progressive approach remains the same: first, help people relax and give them the tools to relax, then help them become familiar with the different aspects of their being from gross to subtle, so eventually they can experience their essential nature as pure consciousness.

For me, this staged approach has been very helpful – as a student and as a teacher. There's a Vedantic analogy that describes it beautifully: If I wanted you to see a dim star in a sky of thousands, if I simply pointed to the sky and said, "do you see that star?" you would probably have no idea what I was pointing to. But if I started with "do you see that big oak tree... do you see the trunk?" you would likely say, "yes", because it's gross, it's obvious and easy to see. Then I would continue guiding, pointing out more and more subtle things, more difficult to see: "follow the trunk up to the first branch… follow that branch up to the first branch on the left… now, follow that smaller branch up to the second branch on the right… see the fork at the very top of that branch... see the bright star at the tip of that branch?" "It's the star three stars above that one". And finally, you'd be able to see the star I was pointing out. This is my approach to Yoga Nidra. To progressively guide people to become familiar with the various aspects of themselves, from gross to subtle: physical body, then energy body, mind, impressions and intuition, so they can eventually experience the Self as pure consciousness. The beauty is, along the way, there's joy and great benefit in becoming acquainted with the various aspects of themselves.

As with the first book, the scripts are arranged in order, starting at the "trunk" – the 15-minute scripts. These scripts introduce people to the practice of Yoga Nidra, help them relax, and teach skills and mindset for relaxing that they can use anytime. Having the ability to relax is the foundation for any further explorations in Yoga Nidra practice.

From there, the scripts get longer and there are explorations of various aspects of the self. In the longest Yoga Nidra practices in this book, time for silence is provided to allow people the opportunity to drop into the state of consciousness that Swami Veda Bharati describes in his book, *My Experiments with Yoga Nidrā*, as "State 3… cognition of negation". My experience of "That" has saved my life. Remembrance of "That" helps me not get mired in "this" – this dream of waking life. When I remember, I suffer less. And that is my wish for you and all the people you share these scripts with. That it leads you to experience "That", so you suffer less with "this", and instead live in more freedom, peace and joy.

Along the way, don't miss the beautiful highlights! Enjoy the discovery or rediscovery of the various aspects of your being. My approach is to keep moving toward the destination, appreciating all the pleasant experiences along the way, for their beauty and value in and of themselves. It's a path of beauty, wonder and awe that I hope you enjoy and can help others enjoy.

About This Book

This book is a companion to the first *"Yoga Nidra Scripts"* book. It shares many things in common:

- Familiar script structure, phrases and language. In my experience, familiarity creates ease and ease leads to more effortless, deeper relaxation.

- Just the right amount of variety to keep curious minds engaged enough to not wander out of the practice or fall asleep.

- Organization from shorter introductory scripts through to full-length Yoga Nidra practices, so you can guide your participants progressively.

- Scripts of different lengths, for different purposes, with elements from a variety of lineages and styles.

- Simple language, accessible to people unfamiliar with yoga terms and those who've learned English as a second language.

- Invitational language, to remind participants that this is *their* practice, to experience in any way they wish.

- Inclusive cues for all people, whether or not they're comfortable or able to lie in savasana.

- Suggested pre- and post-practices to help you plan fuller, more profound sessions. If you're unfamiliar with any of the suggested practices, you can easily find information with an Internet search.

- Ample space for you to make notes if you wish. Edit to your own voice, omit or add elements, as you like – even *I* don't read these scripts the same way twice!
- Approximate timings for the scripts, and suggestions for pauses. When you see: (pause), take a deep breath. When you see: (long pause), take three deep breaths. When you see: (pause for settling) give time until you see your participants moving less, settling into stillness.

Hear samples of the pacing I use with these

FREE audio recordings:

- Anytime Calming
- Overflowing Heart Yoga Nidra
- Rainbow Light Yoga Nidra

Get them at tamaraskyhawk.com/free

Tips for Leading Yoga Nidra

For me, leading a Yoga Nidra session is like doing a verbal dance – an energetic experience of ebb and flow, expressing freely in the moment. Allow inspiration to guide you.

A tip I always give in my Yoga Nidra Teacher Training is to not simply read the scripts, but to experience them yourself, as you're leading the practice. For example, if the script says, "take a breath", then *you* take a breath. If it says, "listen for distant sounds", then *you* listen for distant sounds as well. And so on. This way, you'll not only give the right pacing, you'll also be feeling the intention of the script yourself, getting into the flow and experience of it. Your reading will be less mechanical and much more rich.

Another important tip for leading these Yoga Nidra practices: always remember to serve. You're taking people into deeply-felt experiences – so treat each participant with tender loving care. Who's with you and what do they need? *Ask them.* Choose a script you think might be best. Make sure you've read it, know the content and know whether it's an introductory or intermediate script. Tell them about it. Then ask: "does that sound good?" If there's any hesitation, adjust.

I wish you, and the people you share these Yoga Nidra practices with, much peace, joy and discovery.

Anytime Comfort *(15 min.)*

A quick, comforting practice, like a big, warm hug.

Suggested Pre- and Post-Practices:

- Use before or after a yoga class or other healing treatment. Or if using as a standalone practice, consider beginning with seated shoulder rolls, twists, side bends and forward folds. Comforting, grounding poses such as child's pose, makarasana and squatting poses can also be useful.

- Prepare with a few minutes of a Ganesha Mudra, held at the heart, to stimulate courage, warmth, self care.

- Prepare with deep diaphragmatic breathing to stimulate the relaxation response.

Settling

Getting into a cozy, soothing position. It could be lying on your back, or maybe for this practice, consider lying on your side, hugging a bolster or cushion… or maybe lying on your abdomen… or sitting supported, slightly reclined if possible, with a pillow resting on your chest if it feels comforting.

Choosing *any* position that feels soothing and warm. Getting ready for this practice for comforting.

Tucking a pillow or folded blanket under your head if you like.

Cover yourself with a blanket if it feels warm and cozy.

You know what feels comforting for you. So go ahead and set that up for yourself now. Getting comfy in your own way. Honouring whatever your body needs. (long pause for settling)

Now do a check in. Are your body or mind asking for anything else? If so, answer the call, and give yourself exactly what you need. (pause)

Take a deep breath in now, and as you exhale, feel yourself settling in to the comfort you've created for yourself. (pause)

This practice is just for you. To experience in any way you like.

There is no right or wrong.

You cannot fail. You cannot make a wrong move.

Your experience is perfect just as it is.

Perfect in each moment, as it beautifully unfolds. (pause)

Allowing yourself to sink into the support beneath you. The loving embrace of the earth. Warm, solid, steady support.

Holding you unconditionally.

Letting go into that unconditional embrace of the earth.

The body rests.

Cozy and secure in the sweet comfort.

Just for you.

The body rests, peacefully.

While the awareness continues on.

Free and effortless. (pause)

Yoga Nidra has now begun. (pause)

Rotation of Consciousness

Now moving awareness through the body, freely and effortlessly.

As you move awareness, you *automatically* give the sweet gift of your attention.

If you like, imagine you're giving a quick kiss or smile of attention to each body part.

Your body receives this gift of your attention and feels comforted by it.

The simple, powerful gift of your attention, bringing comfort through the whole body.

Begin with awareness of the right hand

Hello, right hand thumb

Index finger

Middle finger

Ring finger

Little finger

Moving over to the left hand thumb

Quick kiss or smile of attention to the index finger

Middle finger

Ring finger

Little finger

And now shift awareness to the right wrist

Left wrist

Right elbow

Left elbow

Right shoulder

Left shoulder

Hollow of the throat

Travelling up to the back of the head near the top

Crown of the head

Eyebrow centre

Right eyebrow

Left eyebrow

Right eye

Left eye

Right ear

Left ear

Right cheek
Left cheek
Tip of the nose
Upper lip
Lower lip
Chin
Hollow of the throat
The heart centre
Navel centre
Right hip
Left hip
Right knee
Left knee
Right ankle
Left ankle
Right big toe
Second toe
Third toe
Fourth toe
Little toe
Left big toe
Second toe
Third toe
Fourth toe
Little toe
Awareness of the whole right side of the body
The whole right side of the body, comforted by your attention
Awareness of the whole left side of the body
The whole left side of the body, comforted by your attention

Awareness of the whole body together

The whole body together

The whole body together (pause)

Held in the hug of your own loving attention. (long pause)

Breath Awareness/Visualization

Become aware of the support beneath you.

The unconditional support of the earth beneath you. (long pause)

Now become aware of the breath.

The natural breath.

Just as it is.

No need to make any changes, simply watching. (long pause)

Notice with each inhale, you are held in the open arms of the earth.

With each exhale, still held by the earth, unconditionally.

Each inhale, held in the open arms of the earth.

Each exhale, still held by the earth, unconditionally. (long pause)

At every moment, without fail, the earth is here for you.

To hold you when you need a hug.

Solid, steady, strong as a rock.

If it's comforting, you can come back to this feeling of unconditional support from the earth, any time you like.

If it feels good, for the next minute, return to noticing that with each inhale, you are held in the open arms of the earth.

With each exhale, still held by the earth, unconditionally.

Solid support, ever present, that you can return to anytime you like. (pause for 1 minute)

Externalization

Now bring awareness back to the body. (pause)

Take a deep breath.

Feeling awareness rising to the surface. (pause)

Take another deep breath.

Feeling awareness rising to the surface even more. (pause)

Yoga Nidra is now complete. (pause)

Feel your whole body – legs, arms, back, head, resting on the surface beneath you. (pause)

Notice my voice in the room. (pause)

Notice yourself in the room. (pause)

Wiggle your fingers and toes.

Maybe hug your knees into your chest if you're lying down, and rock around.

Stretch or move however you like. (pause)

And if you're lying down, when you're ready, roll to your right side. Take a few deep breaths here. Recalling any experiences of comfort from your practice today. (long pause)

If you were lying down, keeping your eyes closed if you can, slowly press yourself up to sitting. (long pause)

We'll finish by chanting Om three times and Shanti three times. You can join in if you like or simply enjoy the soothing vibration of the sounds.

Taking a deep breath in... Om Om Om Shanti Shanti Shanti (pause)

Carrying the sensation of comfort with you, softly open your eyes.

Anytime Tension Release *(15 min.)*

The perfect practice to release tension after a heavy day of work, study or social engagements.

Suggested Pre- and Post-Practices:

- Prepare with asanas or functional movements that move the spine in all ways – forward, back, twisting, to the side, but avoiding inversion.
- Prepare or finish with self-massage on shoulders, neck, scalp, jaw.
- Prepare or finish with the universal mantra, Om.
- A nice addition to a restful bedtime routine.

Settling

Getting ready to leave tension behind.

Lying in savasana or sitting supported.

If you're lying down and have any tension in the low back, place a pillow or bolster under your knees, maybe something soft under your heels.

Choosing something soft to support and cradle your neck and head.

If you're sitting, reclining slightly if possible.

Maybe choose a scarf or light eye pillow over your eyes or forehead if you're experiencing a headache.

Listening in to your body to hear what it's asking for, then without hesitation, answering the call, giving your body exactly what it needs and deserves.

Your body does so much for you. All day long, every day. And each day, it deserves its well-earned breaks. To take a pause. Rest. Release any built-up tensions. To relax.

Rest, and relax. (pause)

If there's so much tension it's hard to relax, that's fine too. You're welcome just as you are. Simply do your best to create as much comfort as you can, in any way you like. (pause)

And now taking a final scan of the body. Being aware of any areas that feel dull, heavy, tight, irritated. Is there any adjustment you could make to create more comfort? If so, then go ahead and do that now. (pause)

You can't overdo the comfort. There's no prize for doing without an extra cushion, blanket or other prop. This is the all-you-can-comfort buffet. The more you partake, the better you will feel. (pause)

Making any final adjustments now. Settling into the comfort. (pause)

Take a deep breath in, and as you exhale, surrendering to gravity.

Taking another deep breath in, and exhale, release into the comfort.

There is nothing left to do now.

These are moments set aside for rest.

Simply to rest. (pause)

Yoga Nidra has now begun. (pause)

Rotation of Consciousness

Allow awareness to move to the top of the head. The top of the scalp.

Like a cascade, allow tension to be released, from the top of the scalp, down through the rest of the scalp.

A cascade of tension release.

Visualize a cascade of tension release, down from the top, all the way down.

Feel a cascade of tension release.

Now bring awareness to your forehead.

Soften the forehead. Feel awareness expand, from the centre of the forehead, out to the temples.

Softening from the centre of the forehead, out to the temples.

Bring awareness to the eyebrows.

The inside corners of the eyebrows.

Feel awareness expand out, tracing the line of the eyebrows out toward the temples. Softening, widening across the eyebrows.

Bring awareness to the jaw.

Allow the jaw to drop. Soften.

The tongue.

Drop. And soften.

The neck – from the base of the skull, down to the shoulders, softening, lengthening.

Sides and back of the neck, softening, lengthening.

The shoulders – dropping, softening.

The shoulders – dropping and softening. Surrendering to the support.

And now once again, back up to the top of the head. The top of the scalp.

Like a cascade, allow tension to be released, from the top of the scalp, down.

Tension draining from the head.

Awareness moving to the forehead.

Softening the forehead. Expand across the forehead, out to the temples.

Widening across the forehead.

Bring awareness to the eyebrows.

The inside corners of the eyebrows.

Feel awareness expand out, softening, widening across the eyebrows.

Bring awareness to the jaw.

Softening and dropping the jaw.

The tongue.

Dropping and softening.

The neck – from the base of the skull, down to the shoulders, softening, lengthening.

Sides and back of the neck, softening, lengthening.

The shoulders – dropping, softening.

Shoulders on out to the arms, wrists, hands, softening.

The shoulders – dropping and softening. Surrendering to the support.

And now, a cascade of release down the back – between the shoulder blades, release, past the ribs, softening, down to the lower back, cascade of warmth and softening. Pooling at the lower back, a cascade of warmth and soothing.

And now a rush of release, cascading down through the hips, through the legs, to the toes. Like a waterfall of release. Down, and out through the toes.

Now moving awareness back to the top of the head.

Cascade of release, like a waterfall, from the crown of the head, down through the whole body and out through the fingers and toes.

Waterfall of tension release, from the crown down through the whole body, tension released through the fingers and toes.

Tension released from the whole body, out through the fingers and toes.

If it feels good, continue to feel this cascade of release.

Or if you're ready, settle into the calm after the cascade is complete.

Resting peacefully here, for a minute.

Breath Awareness

Now become awareness of the natural breath.

No need to do anything. Simply be aware the natural breath.

With every inhale, know that you are effortlessly drawing in energy. (pause)

Every inhale, effortlessly drawing in energy. (long pause)

With every exhale, feel that you release any remaining tension, as if it's draining away, down and out. (pause)

Every exhale, any remaining tension drains down and out. (pause)

Tension draining, down and out. (long pause)

Continue to be aware of any remaining tension draining out, or if all tension has already dispersed, rest in the effortless peace of the body breathing itself. (pause for several breaths)

Externalization

Ommmmmm

If your mind has wandered off, that's fine. Simply bring awareness back to the breath.

Take a deep breath in and out, feeling awareness rising to the surface, of a body that's feeling less tense than before.

Yoga Nidra is now complete. (pause)

Wiggle your fingers and toes, gently and softly.

Take great care to treat your body kindly.

With love, stretch or move your body however you like. Listening to your body and being kind to allow it whatever it needs. (pause)

And if you're lying down, when you're ready, roll to your right side. Take a few deep breaths here. Recalling any experiences of tension release from your practice today. (long pause)

If you were lying down, keeping your eyes closed if you can, gently press yourself up to sitting. (long pause)

We'll finish by chanting Om three times and Shanti three times. You can join in if you like or simply enjoy the soothing vibration of the sounds.

Taking a deep breath in... Om Om Om Shanti Shanti Shanti (pause)

Using this technique again anytime you need to release tension.

When you're ready, softly open your eyes.

Anytime Soothing *(15 min.)*

A quick practice to help you send energy to any dull or irritated areas.

* This is not a substitute for proper medical care with a qualified doctor.

Suggested Pre- and Post-Practices:

- Prepare with asanas or functional movements that move the spine in all ways – forward, back, twisting, to the side and inverted if possible.
- Prepare or finish with a few minutes of Samana Mudra for calming, soothing, and balancing prana and elemental energies.
- Prepare or finish with a prana-giving mantra such as:

   Om Haum Joom Saha

Settling

Making yourself comfortable for this practice for soothing.

Lying down comfortably on your back, side or abdomen, or sitting up, supported.

Choosing any props you need to feel comfortable – blankets, cushions, bolsters – whatever you need.

Setting yourself up for sublime comfort. So comfortable you won't want to move. Pull out all the stops for ultimate comfort.

If there's an area of tension or discomfort you want to address in this practice today, take extra special care to make sure that area is well supported.

Doing all the things you need to do now, to create comfort. If there are areas of tension preventing you from feeling comfortable or relaxed, that's ok. Welcome those areas just as they are and simply do your best to take good care of them, creating as much comfort and support as possible. (long pause for settling)

Check that your head and neck are as comfortable as possible... jaw softening... shoulders softening... upper back and lower back softening... hips... legs... entire body softening into the support.

Feel the support of the surface beneath you. Let it hold you as you completely surrender to gravity. (pause)

Letting go into the steady support. (pause)

Take a deep breath in... and as you exhale, let go of anything you think you need to do right now. (pause)

There is nothing you need to do. Nothing you have to think about. Set everything aside. (pause)

Bring all of your attention inward. (pause)

Inhale feeling present in this moment.

Exhale letting go of anything outside of this moment.

Inhale feeling present in this moment.

Exhale letting go of anything outside of right here, right now. (pause)

Allowing the body to settle into the ease of non-doing.

Effortless.

Effortless.

Effortless. (pause)

Yoga Nidra has now begun. (pause)

Rotation of Consciousness

Now moving awareness, with ease and effortlessness through the energy centres or chakras.

There's nothing you need to know. No goal or task. Simply be aware of the area when it's mentioned, then allow awareness to freely shift to the next area.

Start with awareness of the point between the eyebrows

Energetic awareness of the point between the eyebrows

Effortless awareness

The point between the eyebrows

The hollow of the throat

Experiencing energetically

The hollow of the throat

The hollow of the throat

The heart centre

Effortless

The heart centre

The heart centre

The navel centre

The navel centre

The navel centre

Moving awareness to the lower abdomen or sacrum

The lower abdomen or sacrum

The lower abdomen or sacrum

Just beyond the tip of the tailbone

Just beyond the tip of the tailbone

Just beyond the tip of the tailbone

Back up to the lower abdomen or sacrum

The lower abdomen or sacrum

The lower abdomen or sacrum

The navel centre

The navel centre

The navel centre
The heart centre
The heart centre
The heart centre
The hollow of the throat
The hollow of the throat
The hollow of the throat
The point between the eyebrows
The point between the eyebrows
The point between the eyebrows
The crown of the head
The crown of the head
The crown of the head

Breath Awareness

Become aware of your breath. Your natural breath. No need to do anything. Simply watching. (pause)

Notice the softness of the breath. (pause)

Air moving softly through the nostrils. (long pause)

Abdomen and chest naturally moving like a gentle wave. (long pause)

Be aware of the softness of your natural breath. (long pause)

Visualization

Now move awareness through the body, physically or energetically, scanning for any area that feels dull, tense, irritated or in any way uncomfortable.

Scanning for any area of discomfort. Simply be aware. (long pause)

If there are multiple areas, choose just one for now. The one that is calling loudest for some soothing. (pause)

As you bring undivided awareness to this area, you bring energy.

Where awareness goes, energy flows. (pause)

Keep awareness on this part, but allow your awareness to become diffused.

Less focused, more diffused, like a cloud of awareness rather than a point.

Diffused, like a cloud of awareness. (long pause)

Feel that as your awareness diffuses, the area of discomfort also disperses and dissolves. (pause)

Irritation, tension, dullness, breaking up. Dispersing. (long pause)

Effortless awareness on the one area.

Diffused.

Discomfort dissolving.

Soothed.

Continue with this diffused awareness, discomfort disappearing. (pause for several breaths)

Now if you like, bring your awareness to one more area that needs soothing.

If there isn't another area, keep awareness on the first area of focus, or bring awareness to the heart centre. (pause)

Effortless, energetic awareness.

Diffused like a cloud.

Feel your effortless awareness diffuse the tension, dullness or blockage of energy.

Diffused awareness, discomfort disappearing. (pause for several breaths)

Externalization

Ommmmmm

And now bringing awareness to your chest.

Inhale, notice your chest rise.

Exhale, notice your chest fall. (pause)

Take a deep breath in and out, feeling awareness rising to the surface, movement breaking up the stillness. (pause)

Yoga Nidra is now complete. (pause)

Feel your whole body – legs, arms, back, head, resting on the surface beneath you. (pause)

Notice my voice in the room. (pause)

Notice yourself in the room. (pause)

Wiggle your fingers and toes.

Stretch or move however you like. (pause)

And if you're lying down, when you're ready, roll to your right side. Take a few deep breaths here. Recalling any experiences of soothing from your practice today. (long pause)

If you were lying down, keeping your eyes closed if you can, slowly press yourself up to sitting. (long pause)

We'll finish by chanting Om three times and Shanti three times. You can join in if you like or simply enjoy the soothing vibration of the sounds.

Taking a deep breath in... Om Om Om Shanti Shanti Shanti (pause)

Using this technique again anytime you need soothing. When you're ready, gently open your eyes.

Anytime Warming *(15 min.)*

A quick practice to warm you up and bring you back to balance on a cold day or whenever you're feeling chilly.

Suggested Pre- and Post-Practices:

- If practicing with a group, check that everyone present will enjoy feeling warmer.
- A soothing practice for people experiencing chilliness or Vata imbalance.
- Prepare with sun salutations to create heat in the body.
- Prepare and/or finish with Surya Bhedana pranayama (breathing), for warming.

Settling

Getting comfortable lying down or sitting supported.

Whichever you choose, having a more closed position can enhance the sensation of warming. For example, keeping the legs and arms closer to the body or the body curled, lying on your side. If it feels good, consider those options. (pause)

Use as many props as you need to feel warmer – sweaters, socks, blankets, *extra* blankets. Cushions and bolsters can also add to the sensation of warmth.

As the body shifts from action to stillness, it naturally cools, so use as many props as you need to make sure you'll stay comfortable throughout the practice.

You'll also want to make sure your head is supported with a cushion or folded blanket for comfort.

Take some time now to get as cozy as you can. Getting comfortable in your own way. (long pause for settling)

Now do a check in. Are your body or mind asking for anything else? If so, answer the call, and give yourself exactly what you need. (pause)

Take a deep breath in now, and as you exhale, feel yourself letting go into the support. (pause)

Sinking in to this cozy support.

Snuggled up.

Relaxing in the knowledge that you've built a cozy set-up, and the longer you stay here, the warmer it will be.

Release tension from the shoulders. (pause)

Release tension from the jaw. (pause)

Knowing with certainty that the warmth is increasing with every breath.

Each breath, feel your body release tension, expanding into that cozy cocoon of increasing warmth. (long pause)

Body supported, bundled.

Body can rest.

Warming beginning.

Awareness continues on. (pause)

Yoga Nidra has now begun. (pause)

Rotation of Consciousness

Now moving awareness through the body.

Awareness moving from point to point, effortlessly.

Start with awareness of the point between the eyebrows

Effortless awareness of the point between the eyebrows

The hollow of the throat

The right shoulder joint

The right elbow joint
Wrist joint
The right thumb
Tip of the index finger
Tip of the middle finger
Tip of the ring finger
Tip of the little finger
The right wrist joint
Elbow joint
Shoulder joint
Hollow of the throat
Shifting to the left shoulder joint
Elbow joint
Wrist joint
The left thumb
Tip of the index finger
Tip of the middle finger
Tip of the ring finger
Tip of the little finger
The left wrist joint
Elbow joint
Shoulder joint
Hollow of the throat
The heart centre (pause)
The hollow of the throat (pause)
The point between the eyebrows (pause)
The tip of the nose (pause)
Resting awareness at the tip of the nose (pause)

Breath Awareness

Become aware of the breath.

The breath in the nostrils. (pause)

No need to change the breath in any way, simply watching the breath.

Notice on the exhalation, warm air going out from the nostrils.

Warm air, moving through the nostrils with each exhalation.

Expansion of the nostrils, and warm air moving through. (pause)

Move awareness to just the right nostril.

Feel as if warmth is generated, each time you breathe in through the right nostril. (long pause)

Follow an inhalation through the right nostril and as you exhale, feel that you exhale through the left nostril.

Inhale warming through the right nostril, exhale out the left nostril.

Inhale warming through the right, exhale out the left.

Warming through and through.

Warmth in the right, and out the left.

If it feels relaxed and easy, keep watching the breath in this way. Or if you prefer, simply focus on the right nostril. (long pause)

Opposites

Now if it feels ok, for just a moment, shift awareness back to the sensation of cold in the body. (pause)

You might feel this as chilliness of the skin... a cold nose, cold cheeks, cold fingers or toes or a sensation of a retraction or contraction, goosebumps.

Noticing any sensations of cold. (pause)

Bringing the sensation of cold to the surface of your awareness.

Really feel the sensation of cold. Tingly, contracting, icy.

And now, let go of the sensation of cold.

Let go of the sensation of cold.

If you're not able to, that's fine. Moving on, to manifest the sensation of heat in the body.

Feel heat arising from deep within your body.

Heat radiating to the surface from the warm core of your body.

Like heat from a blazing fireplace warming up a room – heat from inside your body warming up the space of your body, right out to the surface of the skin, the tips of the fingers, the tips of the toes.

Soothing and warmth radiating from within like a warm cup of tea.

Feel your cheeks flush with warmth.

Getting warmer and warmer.

Heat radiating out, through every pore of your body.

So much heat, sweat is escaping from your pores. Armpits, forehead, eyelids, palms, soles of the feet, gently sweating. Heat throughout the entire body. (pause)

Notice as you're doing this, you have released the sensation of cold.

Noticing that you can manifest the sensation of heat and also release the sensation of cold. You can use this practice to feel warm and cozy anytime you like.

If it feels good, simply continue experiencing the sensation of warmth. (long pause)

Visualization

Now a number of symbols will be mentioned. Images, memories, sensations might arise. As easily as they float into your awareness, allow them to float out. Like clouds in the sky.

Simply watching, with detached awareness.

A roaring fireplace (repeat 3 times)

A fluffy blanket (repeat 3 times)

An ice-capped mountain (repeat 3 times)

A hot bath (repeat 3 times)

A blue moon (repeat 3 times)

A tropical beach (repeat 3 times)

Mid-day sun (repeat 3 times)

Holding awareness of mid-day sun. Radiant, hot, energizing, inviting. (long pause)

Externalization

Now bring awareness back to the breath.

Back to the nostrils.

Feel warm air going out. (pause)

Feel warmth in the nostrils.

Take a deep breath and feel awareness coming back to the body.

Awareness coming back to the body, holding the sensation of warmth.

Yoga Nidra is now complete. (pause)

Feel your whole body – legs, arms, back, head, resting on the surface beneath you. (pause)

Notice yourself in the room. (pause)

Wiggle your fingers and toes.

Stretch your body however you like. If you're lying down, maybe hug your knees into your chest or rock around on your back. (pause)

And also if you're lying down, when you're ready, roll to your right side. Take a few deep breaths here. Remembering any experiences or reflections you would like to hold onto from your practice today. (long pause)

If you were lying down, keeping your eyes closed if you can, slowly press yourself up to sitting. (long pause)

We'll finish by chanting Om three times and Shanti three times.

Taking a deep breath in... Om Om Om Shanti Shanti Shanti (pause)

Carrying any sensations of warmth with you, when you're ready, softly open your eyes.

Anytime Cooling *(15 min.)*

A quick practice to cool you down and bring you back to balance on a hot day or whenever you're feeling overheated.

Suggested Pre- and Post-Practices:

- If practicing with a group, check that everyone present will enjoy feeling cooler.
- A soothing practice for people experiencing hot flashes or Pitta imbalance.
- Prepare and/or finish with Sitali pranayama (breathing), for cooling.
- If preparing with movement or yoga poses, avoid heat-producing practices such as sun salutations or strengthening movements/poses. Opt for gentle stretches, particularly ones that are seated and wide-legged, without the arms raising overhead.

Settling

Getting comfortable lying down or sitting supported.

Whichever you choose, having the arms away from the body and feet apart can enhance the sensation of cooling. If it feels good, consider those options. (pause)

Rather than adding props like blankets, for *this* practice you might want to reduce heat by rolling up your sleeves or pant legs.

You'll want to make sure your head is supported with a cushion or folded blanket for comfort.

Getting comfortable in your own way. (long pause for settling)

Now do a check in. Are your body or mind asking for anything else? If so, answer the call, and give yourself exactly what you need. (pause)

Take a deep breath in now, and as you exhale, feel yourself letting go of tension. (pause)

As the body shifts from action to stillness, it naturally cools.

Feel your body naturally shifting from action to stillness, making way for cooling. (pause)

Releasing into the support beneath you.

Shifting from action to stillness.

Body rests.

Cooling beginning.

Awareness continues on.

Free and effortless. (pause)

Yoga Nidra has now begun. (pause)

Rotation of Consciousness

Now moving awareness through the body.

Awareness moving from point to point, effortlessly.

Start with awareness of the point between the eyebrows

Effortless awareness of the point between the eyebrows

The hollow of the throat

The right shoulder joint

The right elbow joint

Wrist joint

The right thumb

Tip of the index finger

Tip of the middle finger

f the ring finger

Tip of the little finger

The right wrist joint

Elbow joint

Shoulder joint

Hollow of the throat

Shifting to the left shoulder joint

Elbow joint

Wrist joint

The left thumb

Tip of the index finger

Tip of the middle finger

Tip of the ring finger

Tip of the little finger

The left wrist joint

Elbow joint

Shoulder joint

Hollow of the throat

The heart centre (pause)

The hollow of the throat (pause)

The point between the eyebrows (pause)

The tip of the nose (pause)

Resting awareness at the tip of the nose (pause)

Breath Awareness

Become aware of the breath.

The breath in the nostrils. (pause)

No need to change the breath in any way, simply watching the breath.

Notice on the inhalation, cool air coming in through the nostrils.

Cool air, streaming in through the nostrils with each inhalation.

Contraction of the nostrils, and cool air streaming in.

Move awareness to just the left nostril.

Feel cool air coming in through the left nostril, with each inhalation. (long pause)

Follow an inhalation through the left nostril and as you exhale, feel that you exhale through the right nostril.

Inhale cool air through the left nostril, exhale warm air from the right nostril.

Cool air streaming in the left, warm air going out the right.

Cooling the body through the breath.

Cool air in the left nostril, warm air out the right.

If it feels relaxed and easy, keep watching the breath in this way. Or if you prefer, simply focus on the left nostril. (pause for 30 seconds to 1 minute)

Opposites

Now if it feels ok, for just a moment, shift awareness back to the sensation of heat in the body. (pause)

You might feel this as warmth of the skin… a flush in the cheeks… maybe sweat on the palms, feet, eyelids, forehead, or the feeling of an internal fire.

Noticing any sensations of heat. (pause)

Bringing the sensation of heat to the surface of your awareness.

Really feel the sensation of heat. Prickly, expanding. Hot.

And now, let go of the sensation of heat.

Let go of the sensation of heat.

If you're not able to, that's fine. Moving on, to manifest the sensation of cold in the body.

Start by feeling the sensation of a cool breeze blowing across your whole body.

Feel cool air blowing, from your toes all the way up to your face.

Cool, fresh, tingly. Notice the sensations of cold.

Feel your whole body naturally contracting, pulling in from the cold. (pause)

Goosebumps. Shivering. (pause)

Cool like crisp air, cold water, ice.

Feel cold in the body. (long pause)

Notice as you're doing this, you have released the sensation of heat.

Noticing that you can manifest the sensation of cold and also release the sensation of heat. You can use this practice to feel cool and comfortable anytime you like.

If it feels good, simply continue experiencing the sensation of coolness. (long pause)

Visualization

Now a number of symbols will be mentioned. Images, memories, sensations might arise. As easily as they float into your awareness, allow them to float out. Like clouds in the sky.

Simply watching, with detached awareness.

Ice cubes (repeat 3 times)

A sparkling pool (repeat 3 times)

A wood-burning fireplace (repeat 3 times)

Snowflakes falling from the sky (repeat 3 times)

A puffy winter coat (repeat 3 times)

An ice-capped mountain (repeat 3 times)

A blue moon (repeat 3 times)

Holding awareness of a blue moon. Tranquil glow of moonlight. Calming. Cooling. Quenching. (long pause)

Externalization

Now bring awareness back to the breath.

Back to the nostrils.

Feel cool air coming in, and warm air going out. (long pause)

Feel cool air coming in through the nostrils. (pause)

Take a deep breath and feel awareness coming back to the body.

Awareness coming back to the body, holding the sensation of coolness. (pause)

Yoga Nidra is now complete. (pause)

Feel your whole body – legs, arms, back, head, resting on the surface beneath you. (pause)

Notice yourself in the room. (pause)

Wiggle your fingers and toes.

Stretch your body however you like. (pause)

And if you're lying down, when you're ready, roll to your right side. Take a few deep breaths here. Remembering any experiences or reflections you would like to hold onto from your practice today. (long pause)

If you were lying down, keeping your eyes closed if you can, slowly press yourself up to sitting. (long pause)

We'll finish by chanting Om three times and Shanti three times.

Taking a deep breath in... Om Om Om Shanti Shanti Shanti (pause)

Carrying any cooled sensation with you, when you're ready, gently open your eyes.

Permission to Rest *(20 min.)*

Feel good about taking rest when the body or mind is asking for rest.

Suggested Pre- and Post-Practices:

- Use before or after a yoga class or other healing treatment. Or if using as a standalone practice, consider beginning with a simple seated sequence of movements to release tension, such as shoulder rolls, neck stretches, spinal twists, side bends and forward folds.
- Prepare with a few minutes of Abhaya Mudra to calm the mind and stimulate openness.
- Prepare with deep diaphragmatic breathing to stimulate the relaxation response.

Settling

Getting comfortable, lying down or sitting, supported.

Choose any position that feels good right now. Getting ready for this practice to help you feel good about resting, whenever you need rest.

If it feels good, tuck a thin pillow or folded blanket under your head, cover yourself with a blanket, tuck a cushion or bolster under your knees – whatever will help you feel comfortable.

You might choose some of those things, all of them, different things, none of them, all are fine.

This is *your* practice and you know best how to create comfort for you.

So take the time to get comfy now. (long pause for settling)

Notice how the body responds to comfort. You might experience it as a softening, a release, a sinking in or settling. Any way you experience it is welcome.

Checking in with yourself, adjusting as you need. Are your feet feeling that experience of comfort? (pause) What about the legs? (pause) The hips? (pause) The back? (pause) Allow the arms and shoulders to settle into comfort. (pause) The neck. (pause) Jaw. (pause) Forehead. (pause)

Notice the sensations of comfort. (long pause)

Notice – have any thoughts arisen, disturbing your peace or comfort?

Maybe thoughts of your day, expectations, your to-do list, negative self talk – notice any thoughts disrupting the comfort. (pause)

Know that you can choose to let them go in this moment. These thoughts are not needed for the next 20 minutes. You can come back to them after the practice if you like.

For now, you can allow them to melt away, melting into the surface beneath you.

Feel the weight and grip of the thoughts leave you as they melt away. (long pause)

With the mind free from the grip of those thoughts, it's free to enjoy the sensations of comfort.

Notice, in the absence of those thoughts, there is peace. (pause)

Settling into that peace and comfort will be very restorative for you. The more you let go of them now, the more refreshed you will feel, and if you wish, you'll have more energy and presence of mind to process those thoughts after the practice.

But for right now, there's nothing you need to do.

Nothing to accomplish. (pause)

Nothing you need to think about.

Give yourself full permission to simply *be*. (pause)

Just for now, simply being.

Bring awareness to the sweet sensation of comfort. (pause)

Softening into the comfort.

Take a deep breath in… and as you exhale, shift from doing to *being*. (pause)

Take a deep breath in… and as you exhale, shift from thinking to *feeling*. (pause)

Shifting from thinking and doing to feeling and being.

This is your opportunity to simply enjoy peace. (pause)

Make any final adjustments if you haven't already. (pause)

Begin to experience the non-doing even more. Noticing the sensations of comfort, the stillness. Know that you can move, but if it feels good, allow yourself to enjoy this stillness. (pause)

You've done so much, you *do* so much. This is your chance to rest. Simply rest.

This chance for restoration.

Doing nothing. Resting. And gaining everything – peace, comfort, renewed energy, creativity, strength.

It all comes through rest.

Resting now, just as you like. (pause)

Even the mind can rest now.

In its place, there is effortless awareness. (pause)

Feel all experience becoming more and more effortless.

Tranquil and effortless. (pause)

Yoga Nidra has now begun. (pause)

Sankalpa

If it feels right, setting yourself up to enjoy more of this effortless, guilt-free, restorative rest by setting an intention. If you like, mentally repeating:

"When I need to rest, I rest." (pause)

"When I need to rest, I rest." (pause)

Taking a moment to feel the freedom and joy in this statement.
"When I need to rest, I rest." (long pause)

Rotation of Consciousness

Now taking awareness on a trip around the body.
Awareness, floating effortlessly from point to point.
Start by floating awareness to the point between the eyebrows
Effortless awareness of the point between the eyebrows
The hollow of the throat
The right shoulder joint
The right elbow joint
Wrist joint
The right thumb
Tip of the index finger
Tip of the middle finger
Tip of the ring finger
Tip of the little finger
Effortless awareness
The right wrist joint
Elbow joint
Shoulder joint
Hollow of the throat
Shifting awareness over to the left shoulder joint
Elbow joint
Wrist joint
The left thumb
Tip of the index finger
Tip of the middle finger

Tip of the ring finger

Tip of the little finger

Shifting freely, to the left wrist joint

Elbow joint

Shoulder joint

Hollow of the throat

The heart centre

The right side of the chest

The heart centre

The left side of the chest

The heart centre

The heart centre

The heart centre

Resting awareness at the heart centre. (pause)

Breath Awareness

Notice here at the heart centre, at the chest, a gentle rise and fall, like a soft wave. (pause)

Nothing for you to do.

The body is gracefully waving, breathing itself.

Just observe this beautiful wave. (long pause)

Now bring awareness to the nostrils. (pause)

Notice here at the nostrils, subtle contraction on inhalation, expansion on exhalation.

Soft closing and opening.

Just observe this graceful movement of the body breathing itself. (long pause)

These are the sublime movements, intricate workings and effortless intelligence of your being.

You are not the doer.

Simply observe this Divine, exquisite dance of your body breathing itself. (long pause)

Allow awareness to revel in the beauty and miraculous quality of this non-doing. (pause for several breaths)

Sankalpa

Now if you like, mentally repeating your intention again, feeling it with even more clarity, knowing it as your new reality:

"When I need to rest, I rest." (pause)

"When I need to rest, I rest." (pause)

Take a moment to feel the freedom and joy in this statement, knowing that freedom and joy as your new reality.

"When I need to rest, I rest." (long pause)

Externalization

Float awareness back to the heart centre.

Notice the heart centre rising on inhalation, falling on exhalation. (pause)

Feel the heart centre rising on inhalation, falling on exhalation. (pause)

Take a deep breath, feeling the movement break up the stillness. (pause)

Notice that as you breathe, the body is moving, but with ease and effortlessness. (pause)

Bring awareness back to your body.

Feel your body peacefully resting. (pause)

Yoga Nidra is now complete. (pause)

Notice your body, surrendered to gravity. (pause)

Be aware of the room, the space around you, the objects. (long pause)

Notice any sounds and how they travel through the space, giving you a sense of the size of the space. (long pause)

Begin to wiggle your fingers and toes, moving against gravity.

Feel yourself more aware of the body now, and the body at ease.

Stretch or move in any way you like. (pause)

If you're lying down, when you're ready, roll to your right side. If you like, repeat your intention one more time: "When I need to rest, I rest." (pause)

If it feels good, know this as your new reality. (long pause)

If you were lying down, keeping your eyes closed, gently press yourself up to sitting. (long pause)

We'll finish by chanting Om three times and Shanti three times.

Take a deep breath in…

Om Om Om Shanti Shanti Shanti (pause)

And before opening your eyes, give yourself a moment of gratitude for allowing yourself this beautiful, restorative, permission to rest.

Inspire & Energize (Kapha Pacifying)
(20 min.)

A practice that can be used by anyone to inspire and energize, but is particularly beneficial for people with abundant Kapha dosha.

Suggested Pre- and Post-Practices:

- Begin with a few gentle sun salutations to loosen up the body.
- Begin with some Kapalabhati pranayama (breathing), to raise some energy toward the mind and prevent sleeping.
- Prepare and/or finish with a prana-giving mantra such as:

   Om Haum Joom Saha
- Also consider finishing with some energizing sun salutations or a playful yoga class to instantly begin the habit of turning inspiration into action.
- Finish with a few minutes of Prana Mudra to harness energy.

Settling

Getting set up in your favourite resting position – on your back, your side, your abdomen, or sitting, supported. Sitting can be a great option if you tend to fall asleep in Yoga Nidra practices. It can be a little assist to staying awake.

Choose any position that feels supportive. (pause)

Getting ready for your Yoga Nidra practice to energize and inspire. Energizing while doing nothing. What could be easier?

Making your body comfortable with any props you need. A thin pillow or folded blanket under your head. If you're lying on your back, maybe a bolster under your knees to support your low back, possibly something under your heels. Taking time to get set up. (long pause for settling)

And now, check in with how you feel.

Your set-up should make you feel at ease, but not sleepy. (pause)

If you do feel sleepy, you could make it slightly less warm, slightly less dark.

You can also check your head position. If your chin is tucked in, it can stimulate sleep. Try reducing the size of the support under your head so your head is in a neutral alignment, chin neither tucked nor raised, and notice how it might change your energy and alertness.

Check that you feel relaxed yet still alert, not sleepy. (pause)

Set yourself up so you can stay awake and aware, in peaceful ease. (pause)

Now that you're supported, begin to feel a sense of ease setting in.

Body is resting.

Beginning the process of turning the senses inward.

Become aware of any scent in the room.

Take deep breaths, noticing any scent in the room. (long pause)

Now picture the room you're in. The ceiling... the walls... anything in the room... the floor... the space directly around you... visualizing. (pause)

Feel the texture of the props you're using. Soft, hard. (pause)

Feel the texture of your clothing – smooth, rough. (long pause)

Be aware of sounds. Become aware of sounds far away. (long pause)

Now be aware of sounds closer in, within the room. (long pause)

Be aware of the closest sound, the sound of your body breathing. (long pause)

Yoga Nidra has now begun. (pause)

Sankalpa

If you have a sankalpa, allow it to arise in your awareness now. If you don't have a sankalpa, you can use the affirmation: "I am energized", or any other statement that feels good. (long pause)

Allow the *feeling* of your sankalpa to grow. Feel it igniting your heart, inspiring and exciting you. (long pause)

With joy, repeat your chosen sankalpa or "I am energized", three times mentally now. (long pause)

You can be certain your sankalpa is already working its magic from deep within you. (pause)

Rotation of Consciousness/Breathing

Now beginning the process of energizing the body.

Bring awareness to the right hand

Fingers, palm

As you inhale, feel that you pull energy in to the right hand

And as you exhale, feel that you release any dullness

Awareness over to the left hand now

Fingers, palm

As you inhale, feel that you pull energy in to the left hand

And as you exhale, feel that you release any dullness

Now over to the right arm

As you inhale, feel that you pull energy in to the right arm

And as you exhale, feel that you release any dullness

Awareness over to the left arm now

Inhale energy

Exhale dullness

Now bring awareness to the chest and abdomen

Inhale energy

Exhale dullness

Now bring awareness to the back

Upper back, mid-back and lower back

Inhale energy

Exhale dullness

Now bring awareness to the right leg

Inhale energy

Exhale dullness

Now bring awareness to the left leg

Inhale energy

Exhale dullness

Bring awareness to the right foot

Inhale energy

Exhale dullness

Bring awareness to the left foot

Inhale energy

Exhale dullness

Now bring awareness all the way up to the tailbone

Lower abdomen

Navel centre

Heart centre

Hollow of the throat

Allow awareness to travel swiftly now. Where awareness goes, energy flows.

Allow awareness to move up the back of the neck to the back of the head near the top

Then up to the crown of the head

Down to the eyebrow centre

Moving swiftly, sweeping energy

Right eyebrow

Left eyebrow

Right eye

Left eye

Right ear

Left ear

Right cheek

Left cheek

Tip of the nose

Upper lip

Lower lip

Tip of the chin

Hollow of the throat

Heart centre

Heart centre

Heart centre (pause)

Now be aware of the whole body together

The whole body together

The whole body relaxed, yet energized

Body in perfect balance (pause)

Welcome the whole body of beautiful light energy, all at once. (pause)

Take a moment to feel the exciting potential of an energized body. (pause)

You can pour this energy into the things you love to do. (pause)

Take a moment to visualize yourself pouring this energy into the things you love. (pause for 30 seconds)

Sankalpa

Now is the perfect time to allow your sankalpa to arise in your awareness again. If you don't have a sankalpa, you can use: "I am energized", or the statement you chose earlier. (pause)

Allow the *feeling* of your sankalpa to grow. Feel it igniting your heart, exciting and inspiring you. (long pause)

With confidence and joy, repeat your sankalpa or "I am energized", three times mentally now. (long pause)

Know with certainty that your sankalpa is already working its magic from deep within you, creating exciting new realities. (pause)

Externalization

Bring awareness back to your energized body.

Feel your body breathing. (pause)

Feel your chest rising and falling. (pause)

Picture the room you're in. The space around you… the floor… the walls… the ceiling. (long pause)

Know that your Yoga Nidra practice is wrapping up.

Take a couple of deep breaths and notice any scent in the room.

Take deep breaths, noticing any scent in the room. (long pause)

Yoga Nidra is now complete. (pause)

Move your body. In any way that feels good. Stretch, roll your ankles and wrists. Maybe draw your knees into your chest if you're lying down. Whatever feels nice. Feel your body coming alive with energy. (long pause)

And if you're lying down, when you're ready, roll to the right side. (pause)

Take a few deep breaths, awareness coming back into your day, holding any sensation of being energized or inspired. (long pause)

Now if you were lying down, move up to sitting. (long pause)

Sitting up, back as straight as you can make it.

Feeling the energy rise as you sit. (pause)

Take a deep breath in… and a long breath out.

If you like, mentally repeat your sankalpa or "I am energized", one more time, to keep it top of mind. (pause)

We'll finish by chanting Om and Shanti, three times each.

Join in if you can. Feel the energy rise with the chant.

Chanting and singing is excellent for raising energy and inspiration.

Take a deep breath in.

Om Om Om Shanti Shanti Shanti (pause)

Ready to channel energy and inspiration into your favourite things, greet the day again by opening your eyes.

Magical Morning *(20-25 min.)*

A magical way to start your day feeling energized, with a positive outlook.

Suggested Pre- and Post-Practices:

- Can be used just after waking or in combination with a morning yoga practice or healing treatment.
- Prepare with a few minutes of Samana Mudra for balancing elemental energies and centering.
- Prepare with Anuloma Viloma pranayama for balancing out Rajas and Tamas (activity and inertia), as well as balancing out the activation of the right and left brain hemispheres.
- Consider diffusing essential oils to set the tone for the morning, as long as all participants are comfortable with the scent.
- Prepare and/or finish with some basic movements of the joints, simple stretches or self-massage to enliven the body.
- Prepare and/or finish with a Shanti Mantra, such as:

    Sarvesham svastir bhavatu

    Sarvesham shantir bhavatu

    Sarvesham purnam bhavatu

    Sarvesham mangalam bhavatu

    (May prosperity be unto all, may peace be unto all, may fullness be unto all, may auspiciousness be unto all)

Settling

Gathering all the props you need to comfortably lie in savasana or sit supported for this Magical Morning practice. (pause)

Maybe a pillow for your head, a blanket to cover you, maybe something for under your knees, an eye pillow, fluffy socks or sweater if you find it a chilly morning. Anything you're going to need to be comfortable. (pause)

If you're feeling sleepy, maybe skip the extra blanket or eye pillow. If it's too warm or dark, it might cause you to fall asleep.

Getting yourself set up for your Yoga Nidra practice, lying down or sitting supported. (long pause for settling)

Now that you're comfortable in your resting position, we'll begin this Magical Morning practice with a few simple stretches. Releasing any tension that might have built up over the night.

If it's comfortable, close your eyes. You'll be guided through these simple movements.

To begin, stretch your arms overhead, stretch your legs out, lengthen the whole body… and release.

Point your toes toward the floor… flex your feet toward your face… and release.

Press your lower back *down* if you're in savasana, *back* if you're sitting… and release.

Lift your chest, squeeze your shoulder blades together… and release.

Shrug your shoulders… press your shoulders down toward your feet… and release.

Make fists. Squeeze them tight… open your fingers wide… and release.

Move your head slowly from side to side… and back to centre.

Tense all of your face toward your nose, make a tight, squished face… and release.

Now open your jaw wide, stick out your tongue and breathe out... haaa

And now, settling in for stillness. Make any adjustments you need now, keeping your eyes closed if you can. (long pause)

Beginning to become aware of the senses. Some suggestions will be made. You might experience your senses, and you might not. Both are fine. There's nothing you need to do, simply witness.

First noticing any scent in the room. Scents in the whole room, scents nearby, the scent within your own nostrils. Noticing any scents. Without analyzing. Simply noticing. (long pause)

Now shifting awareness to taste. Noticing any taste in the mouth. Bitter, sweet, saline... awareness of any taste you might be experiencing. (long pause)

Moving awareness to visualizing. Without opening your eyes, visualize the space you're in – the size... the things nearby... their colour and shapes. Awareness of the surface you're resting on and the objects you're using as props. Visualize their colour, shape, size. (long pause)

Now bring awareness to the texture of the props you're using. *Feel the quality of the textures against your skin... feel the temperature of the air on your cheeks, nose, forehead.* (pause)

And finally, being aware of any sounds. Begin with the furthest sound you can hear. Not analyzing, just noticing. The furthest sound you can hear. (long pause)

Now being aware of any nearby sounds. (long pause)

And finally, the sound of your own breath. Awareness of the soft sound of your body breathing. (long pause)

Yoga Nidra has now begun. (pause)

Rotation of Consciousness/Breathing

Now beginning the process of energizing the body, to prepare for the day ahead.

Bring awareness to the right hand

Fingers, palm, back of the hand, wrist

Noticing the right hand

As you inhale, feel that you pull energy in to the right hand

And as you exhale, feel that you *release* any sensation of dullness or tension

Awareness of the right hand

Inhaling energy

Exhaling any dullness or tension

Awareness over to the left hand now

Fingers, palm, back of the hand, wrist

Noticing the left hand

As you inhale, feel that you pull energy in to the left hand

And as you exhale, feel that you *release* any sensation of dullness or tension

Awareness of the left hand

Inhaling energy

Exhaling any dullness or tension

Now over to the right arm

Lower arm, elbow, upper arm, shoulder

Awareness of the right arm

As you inhale, feel that you pull energy in to the right arm

And as you exhale, feel that you *release* any sensation of dullness or tension

Awareness of the right arm

Inhaling energy

Exhaling any dullness or tension

Awareness over to the left arm now

Lower arm, elbow, upper arm, shoulder

Awareness of the left arm

As you inhale, feel that you pull energy in to the left arm

And as you exhale, feel that you *release* any sensation of dullness or tension

Awareness of the left arm

Inhaling energy

Exhaling any dullness or tension

Now bring awareness to the chest and abdomen

Chest and abdomen

Awareness of the chest and abdomen

As you inhale, feel that you pull energy in to the chest and abdomen

And as you exhale, feel that you *release* any sensation of dullness or tension

Awareness of the chest and abdomen

Inhaling energy

Exhaling any dullness or tension

Now bring awareness to the back

Upper back, mid-back and lower back

Awareness of the back

As you inhale, feel that you pull energy in to the back

And as you exhale, feel that you *release* any sensation of dullness or tension

Awareness of the back

Inhaling energy

Exhaling any dullness or tension

Now bring awareness to the right leg

Hip, thigh, knee, lower leg

Awareness of the right leg

As you inhale, feel that you pull energy in to the right leg

And as you exhale, feel that you *release* any sensation of dullness or tension

Awareness of the right leg

Inhaling energy

Exhaling any dullness or tension

Now bring awareness to the left leg

Hip, thigh, knee, lower leg

Awareness of the left leg

As you inhale, feel that you pull energy in to the left leg

And as you exhale, feel that you *release* any sensation of dullness or tension

Awareness of the left leg

Inhaling energy

Exhaling any dullness or tension

Now bring awareness to the right foot

Ankle, top of the foot, sole of the foot, toes

Awareness of the right foot

As you inhale, feel that you pull energy in to the right foot

And as you exhale, feel that you *release* any sensation of dullness or tension

Awareness of the right foot

Inhaling energy

Exhaling any dullness or tension

Now bring awareness to the left foot

Ankle, top of the foot, sole of the foot, toes

Awareness of the left foot

As you inhale, feel that you pull energy in to the left foot

And as you exhale, feel that you *release* any sensation of dullness or tension

Awareness of the left foot

Inhaling energy

Exhaling any dullness or tension

Now bring awareness all the way up to the navel centre... the heart centre... to the neck and throat

Awareness resting at the neck and throat

Back of the neck, sides of the neck, front of the neck, hollow of the throat

Awareness of the neck and throat

As you inhale, feel that you pull energy in to the neck and throat

And as you exhale, feel that you *release* any sensation of dullness or tension

Awareness of the neck and throat

Inhaling energy

Exhaling any dullness or tension

Now allow awareness to travel swiftly. Where awareness goes, energy follows, like painting a beautiful ribbon of light energy from point to point. Beautiful light energy, sweeping through the head and face.

Allow awareness to travel from the throat, up the back of the neck to the back of the head near the top

Then up to the crown of the head

Down to the eyebrow centre

Beautiful light energy, sweeping from point to point

Right eyebrow

Left eyebrow

Right eye

Left eye

Right ear

Left ear

Right cheek

Left cheek

Tip of the nose

Upper lip

Lower lip

Tip of the chin

Hollow of the throat

Heart centre

Now welcoming the whole body together

The whole body together

The whole body together (pause)

Welcome the whole body of beautiful light energy, all at once. (long pause)

Breath Awareness/Visualization

Noticing this sensation of light within the body

And also become aware of the light surrounding the body

The morning light

Charged with energy and potential

Take a moment to breathe in the morning light with your whole body

Soaking in its energy and potential.

Soaking in the beauty of the morning light with your whole being.

Observing this simple breath for the next minute. Breathing in the beauty, energy and potential of the morning light, with your whole body. (pause for 1 minute)

Externalization

Noticing again, the soft sound of your body breathing. (pause)

Notice any nearby sounds. (long pause)

Notice the texture of the props you're using. *Feel* the quality of the textures against your skin... feel the temperature of the air on your cheeks, nose, forehead. (long pause)

Remembering the space you're in. Visualize the things nearby... their colour and shapes, visualize the size of the space and your body within it. (long pause)

Noticing any taste in the mouth. Bitter, sweet, saline... awareness of any taste you might be experiencing. (long pause)

And finally, noticing any scent in the room. The scent within your own nostrils, scents nearby, the scent of the room. (long pause)

Yoga Nidra is now complete. (pause)

Take a few deep breaths and feel movement coming back to the body.

Awareness coming back to the surface, fresh and ready for a beautiful day ahead. (long pause)

Wiggle your fingers and toes. Feel the lightness of the sensation.

Stretch or move in any way you like. (long pause)

If you're lying down, roll to your right side. Take a moment to appreciate the opportunity to greet the day with any positive sensations that might have arisen in your practice today. (long pause)

If you were lying down, keeping your eyes closed if you can, gently press yourself up to sitting, and take a deep breath in, taking in the morning air, morning light on your face. (long pause)

Once more... deep breath in, taking in the morning air, morning light on your face. (pause)

We'll finish by chanting Om Shanti Shanti Shanti.

Om Shanti Shanti Shanti. (pause)

Open your eyes to greet the beautiful day ahead.

Restful Night *(20-30 min.)*

A peaceful practice to get you ready for a restful night and sweet dreams.

Suggested Pre- and Post-Practices:

- Prepare with stretches for the major muscles to release any tension that's built up during the day. (For example: front and back of thighs, calves, hips, lower back, upper back, shoulders, neck, ankles, wrists, jaw.)

- Prepare with self-massage on shoulders, neck, scalp, jaw, hands and feet.

- Finish with a calming nightly routine that includes anything that helps you feel restful, for example, essential oils, tea, bath.

- This practice has an optional sankalpa section for people with a personal sankalpa. If you'd like to include this, but have participants new to sankalpa, start with a brief explanation or the Guided Sankalpa Setting from the first *Yoga Nidra Scripts* book.

Settling

Getting settled for this practice to help you wind down for the day.

Getting into a comfortable position, sitting supported or lying down, either in savasana or a pose similar to how you usually sleep. Use any cushions or blankets you need. (pause)

The purpose of this practice isn't to put you to sleep but to prepare you for sleep. But, if you happen to fall asleep, that's ok, too. At least you'll know what helped you fall asleep and you can repeat those practices anytime you like, when it's time to sleep. (pause)

Right now, *comfort* is your top priority. For your body to relax enough to fall into sleep, you'll need to create comfort that your body is happy to sink into.

So if you haven't created the most comfortable set-up possible for yourself, go ahead and do that. Adjust any and all of the things you need.

Imagine yourself as a cat, taking time to settle in, smoothing and fluffing the resting place until it's just right, then snuggling in, cozy and relaxed. (long pause for settling)

Snuggling in, for this practice of rest.

Body will sleep, yet awareness will continue on.

Effortless awareness.

Beginning the process of withdrawing the senses. Drawing them inside.

Start by becoming aware of any scent in the room.

Take deep breaths, noticing any scent in the room. (long pause)

And now, scents closer to you. The scent of your clothing… your hair… the scent within your nostrils. (long pause)

Now releasing awareness of scent. (pause)

Visualize your body relaxing. As if you are viewing your body from above. Visualize your body relaxing in the room. See the props… the clothing… the space around you… the objects in the room… the walls… the ceiling… the floor. (pause)

Now releasing awareness of sight. (pause)

Feel the temperature of the air on your face. Your cheeks, your forehead, your nose. (pause)

The temperature of the air moving through your nostrils. Feeling the temperature of the air. (long pause)

Now releasing awareness of touch. (pause)

Be aware of sounds. Listening for the furthest sounds you can hear. (long pause)

Now listening for sounds within the room. (long pause)

And finally, listening for the sound of your own body breathing. (long pause)

Now switching from listening to *hearing*.

Switching from listening, to hearing.

Be effortless.

Activity shifts to *effortlessness*.

Effortless awareness.

Yoga Nidra has now begun. (pause)

> **Optional: Sankalpa**
>
> Now, if you have a sankalpa, allow it to arise in your awareness, along with the joyful feeling of it. (long pause)
>
> Repeat your sankalpa mentally, three times now. (long pause)

Rotation of Consciousness

Now allowing awareness to travel into the body.

Bring awareness to the crown of the head.

Be aware of the scalp, the tissue of the scalp.

Then move awareness down, into the bone of the skull at the crown of the head.

Awareness moving down through the bone of the skull, over the slope of the forehead to the bone between the eyebrows

Down through the bones around the eyes to the cheekbones

Out toward the joint of the jaw

Following the jawline, down to the tip of the chin

Back up to the crown of the head

Awareness moving through the bone, down the back of the skull to the base of the skull

Moving into the top of the spine

Moving down through the vertebrae of the neck

And over to the right shoulder joint

Awareness moving like warm molasses, down, through the centre of the right upper arm bone

Through the elbow joint

Down, through the lower arm bones

To the wrist joint

Down, through the bones of the right thumb

The bones of the index finger

Middle finger

Ring finger

Little finger

Awareness retracting back up through the finger bones, to the wrist, through the bones of the lower arm, elbow joint and upper arm bone, back to the shoulder

Awareness moving through the right collarbone

Hopping over the hollow of the throat

Over to the left collarbone, out to the left shoulder joint

Awareness moving like warm molasses, down, through the centre of the left upper arm bone

Through the elbow joint

Down, through the lower arm bones

To the wrist joint

Down, through the bones of the left thumb

The bones of the index finger

Middle finger

Ring finger

Little finger

Awareness retracting back up through the finger bones, to the wrist, through the bones of the lower arm, elbow joint and upper arm bone, back to the shoulder

Awareness moving through the left collarbone toward the hollow of the throat

And now back to the top of the spine at the base of the skull

Moving down the vertebrae of the neck, to the upper back

Awareness of the shoulder blades

Awareness of the rib bones, curling out from the spine around to the front

Awareness back to the spine, moving through the vertebrate of the middle back, then lower back

To the sacrum, through the sacrum to the tailbone

Then following the pelvis around to the right and left hip joints

Awareness travelling down, like warm molasses, deep in the centre of the upper leg bones, through the knee joints, down through the bones of the lower legs to the ankles, the heels, the bones of the feet, down through the bones of the big toes, second toes, third toes, fourth toes, little toes. (long pause)

Breath Awareness

Now bring awareness to the ribcage. Notice the ribcage expanding and contracting as your body breathes.

No need to make any changes to the breath.

Simply noticing the natural expansion and contraction of the ribcage as your body breathes. (long pause)

Now bring awareness to the air moving in and out of the body.

Follow the air as it moves in through the nostrils, down to the lungs, and follow the air as it moves up and out through the nostrils.

Follow the movement of the air.

Watching the air. (long pause)

Continue watching the air.

The subtle quality of the air, as it moves in and out of the body.

Awareness of the subtle quality of the air. (long pause)

Now allowing awareness to dissolve, into the *space* in which the air is moving.

Awareness dissolving, into the *space* in which the air is moving.

The space inside the body. (pause)

The space around the body. (pause)

Allow awareness to dissolve into the subtlest quality, of space. (pause)

Awareness dissolving into space.

The quality of space. Still. Effortless. All-pervading, space. (long pause)

If it feels peaceful, allow awareness to rest now in this quality of still, effortless space for the next several minutes. (pause for 4-10 min.)

> **Optional: Sankalpa**
>
> Now allow your sankalpa to arise once again in your consciousness, along with the joy that it brings. (long pause)
>
> Repeat your sankalpa mentally, three times now. (long pause)
>
> Know that your sankalpa is now nestled in a deep part of your consciousness, already working its magic on all aspects of your being, positively affecting all of your future actions. (long pause)

Externalization

Now bring awareness back to the breath. (pause)

Noticing the soft movement of air, in and out of the nostrils. (pause)

Be aware of the ribcage expanding and contracting with each breath. (pause)

Feel the body resting peacefully. (pause)

Be aware of the room where the body is resting peacefully.

Visualize the body resting in the room. (pause)

Visualize the room. The floor… the walls… the ceiling. (long pause)

Take a couple of deep breaths, noticing any scent in the room. (long pause)

Feel awareness rising, back into the body, back into the room.

Yoga Nidra is now complete. (pause)

Wiggle your fingers and toes, gently and softly. (pause)

Stretch your body from head to toe. (long pause)

And if you're lying down, roll to your right side. Take a few deep breaths. (long pause)

If you were lying down, keeping your eyes closed if you can, gently press yourself up to sitting. (long pause)

We'll finish by chanting Om three times and Shanti three times. You can join in if you like. Let it be the lullaby to lead you toward a restful sleep.

Taking a deep breath in… Om Om Om Shanti Shanti Shanti (pause)

Have a wonderful evening, a soothing night routine and a beautiful sleep.

Slowly open your eyes when you're ready.

Courageous Confidence *(25 min.)*

Dive deep into the heart of courage and emerge confident, fearless and ready to take on anything.

Suggested Pre- and Post-Practices:

- Prepare and/or finish with some stretches to release tension in the body, emphasizing heart-opening poses and movements.
- Prepare with a few minutes of Abhaya Hridaya Mudra, to stimulate a fearless heart.
- Prepare and/or finish with the mantra, Soham (I am That), to stimulate feelings of connectedness, confidence, limitlessness.

Settling

Getting comfortable – lying on your back or sitting up, supported.

Making a cozy rest nest with any props you need – cushions, blankets, bolsters, eye pillow – whatever you need to feel as comfortable as possible at this time and in this place. (long pause)

Getting ready to do nothing. (pause)

In this practice for courage, you have the opportunity to just rest for a while.

Imagine that. Simply resting.

If it feels good, you can let the body rest, the senses rest, the monkey mind rest – so the heart, the deeper intelligence, and intuition can be heard.

This time is just for you.

To experience in the way you like.

You can't make a wrong move.

There are no shoulds or shouldn'ts you need to hold onto.

You can participate in this experience in any way you like. In any way that feels good.

This is for *you*.

So make yourself as comfortable as you like in just the way you like. Adjusting anything you need, to feel supported, held, and free to let go of tensions. (pause)

Checking that each body part is as relaxed as can be. If you can't completely relax, that's fine. You're welcome just as you are. (pause)

Check that your feet and ankles are relaxed as can be. (pause)

Calves, knees and thighs relaxed as can be. (pause)

Hips relaxed as can be. (pause)

Lower back, middle back, upper back releasing tension. Whole back, melting. (pause)

Hands and arms letting go. (pause)

Shoulders and neck melting, tension diffusing. (pause)

Jaw, tongue and cheeks softening. (pause)

Eyes, forehead and scalp, softening. (pause)

Whole body, melting into the support of the earth beneath you. Held by the support of the earth beneath you. (pause)

Nothing for you to do.

Body is supported and resting. (pause)

Awareness continues on. (pause)

Visualize the room around you. Remembering the details. See the props you're resting on... the space around you... any furniture in the room... walls... doors... windows... the ceiling... the floor. (pause)

Now feel the warmth or coolness of the air on your face. Cheeks, forehead, nose – noticing the temperature of the air. Feeling the temperature of the air. (long pause)

Shifting to hearing now. Hearing sounds far, sounds near – a mesh of sounds. No need to identify. Simply be aware of the mesh of sounds. (pause)

Effortless awareness of sound. (long pause)

Body is resting, mind settling. Only the sense of hearing remains.

You can come back to body awareness and alert senses anytime you like, simply by opening your eyes.

But if it feels good, allow the body to rest, the mind to settle and the senses to turn within.

Effortless.

Awareness continues on.

Awake and aware.

Yoga Nidra has now begun. (pause)

Sankalpa

If you have a sankalpa, allow it to arise in your awareness now. If you don't have a sankalpa, you can use the affirmation: "I am courageous and confident", or any other statement that feels right. (long pause)

Allow the joy of the sankalpa to rise and grow, permeating every part of your being. Personal sankalpa or "I am courageous and confident". (pause)

Feel without a doubt, that the sankalpa is already becoming reality, right at this moment.

With certainty and clarity, repeat your sankalpa or "I am courageous and confident, three times mentally now. (long pause)

Know that this mental impression is now rooted in your being, along with all of the joy it will bring. (pause)

Rotation of Consciousness

Now beginning the process of sweeping awareness through the body.

Effortless awareness, sweeping from one point to the next.

Float awareness over to the right hand

Right hand thumb

Index finger

Middle finger

Ring finger

Little finger

Awareness floating over to the left hand thumb

Index finger

Middle finger

Ring finger

Little finger

Right wrist

Left wrist

Right elbow

Left elbow

Right shoulder

Left shoulder

Hollow of the throat

Back of the head near the top

Crown of the head

Eyebrow centre

Right eyebrow

Left eyebrow

Right eye

Left eye

Right ear

Left ear

Right cheek

Left cheek

Tip of the nose

Upper lip

Lower lip

Tip of the chin

Hollow of the throat

The heart centre

The right side of the chest

The heart centre

The left side of the chest

The heart centre

The heart centre

The heart centre

Awareness resting at the heart centre. (pause)

Breath Awareness/Visualization

Bring awareness to the breath.

The natural breath, nothing for you to do.

Keep awareness at the heart centre and notice the gentle rising and falling of the chest. (pause)

Body is taking care of your breath for you, all by itself.

There's nothing you need to do.

For a moment, simply noticing this miracle of your body undertaking all the complex processes of breathing, with grace and without expectation. (pause)

You are supported by your body.

Cared for by your body.

Every moment of your life.

Your body is doing its best for you.

Taking a moment in gratitude and appreciation for this miracle of your body breathing itself. Knowing just what to do. And doing it without expectation. (pause)

You are supported by this breath at every moment in your life.

Supported by the intelligence behind the breath at every moment in your life.

Supported by the energy fuelling the intelligence, at every moment in your life.

At every moment of your life.

Supported effortlessly, by miraculous intelligence and energy. The wind beneath your wings.

Soar high. Be free. Be bold.

Soar high. Be free. Be bold.

You are supported at every moment by a higher intelligence. Supported effortlessly with energy.

Spread your wings and fly. All the conditions are there. If you falter, the conditions will still be there and you can try again. (pause)

You are always supported by a higher intelligence and energy. There is a current already there to lift you up. Allow the current to lift you, high into the sky, soaring. (pause)

This is the nature of your being. You are always supported by a higher intelligence and energy, at every moment.

The very same intelligence and energy supporting every person, animal, blade of grass.

Experience this connection to higher intelligence, energy, constant support.

Experience this connection in any way you like. Visualizing or feeling... soaring, supported, miraculous potential.

Experience this connection to higher intelligence, energy, constant support in any way you like.

Let it fuel the sensation of effortless confidence and courage. (pause)

Experiencing this in any way you like for the next few minutes. (pause for 2-10 minutes)

Sankalpa

And now, allow your sankalpa to arise in your awareness again.

Allow your sankalpa to arise in your awareness, or if you don't have a sankalpa, use: "I am courageous and confident", or the statement you chose earlier. (long pause)

Allow the joy of the sankalpa to rise and grow, permeating every part of your being. (pause)

Feel without a doubt that the sankalpa is already becoming reality, right at this moment.

With certainty and clarity, repeat your sankalpa or "I am courageous and confident", three times mentally now. (long pause)

Know that this mental impression is now rooted deep in the source of your *destiny*, along with all of the joy it will bring. (pause)

Externalization

Ommmm

Bringing awareness back to the breath. Notice your body breathing. Feel your body breathing. (pause)

Take a moment to enjoy the non-doing of your breathing. (pause)

Now take a deep breath in. Feel energy and awareness coming back into the body. (pause)

Listening for sounds. Being aware of my voice. Listening for sounds in the room, sounds far away. Listening for sounds. (long pause)

Now noticing the warmth or coolness of the air on your face. Cheeks, forehead, nose. Feeling the temperature of the air. (pause)

Remembering the details of the room. See the props you're resting on, the space around you, any furniture, walls, doors, windows, ceiling. (pause)

Awareness coming back into the room, back into your body.

Yoga Nidra is now complete. (pause)

Take a deep breath. (pause)

If you feel like making gentle movements in the body, make them. If you feel like making larger movements, make them. Moving, stretching however you'd like. (pause)

If you were lying down, roll to your right side and take a few breaths, recalling any sensations of courage or other insights you gained in your practice. (long pause)

And now, keeping your eyes closed if you can, trying to disturb the body as little as possible, make your way to sitting upright. (long pause)

Feel the body and mind activating. And yet, still remaining relaxed. (pause)

I'll finish by chanting Om and Shanti three times each.

Join in if you like, then when you're ready, open your eyes, coming fully back to body awareness and alert senses, carrying the sense of confidence and courage.

Take a deep breath in.

Om Om Om Shanti Shanti Shanti (pause)

Fresh Start *(25 min.)*

Connect with your innate freedom and give yourself the permission to refresh, anytime you need.

Suggested Pre- and Post-Practices:

- Begin with a relaxed asana or movement practice that loosens up the joints and major muscles.
- Begin with a few minutes of holding Abhaya Mudra for courage and openness to shift into a new reality. Combine with chanting of Om.
- Set the tone by beginning with the inspiring words of Mahatma Gandhi: "Each night, when I go to sleep, I die. And the next morning, when I wake up, I am reborn." At any moment, we have the opportunity to start fresh.
- Finish with Breath of Joy pranayama and self-massage on the shoulders, back of the neck, scalp, arms, legs and soles of the feet.

Settling

Finding a comfortable place to lie down, or sit up, supported.

Getting ready for this practice to help you open up to a fresh start. (pause)

Support your head and neck with a thin pillow or folded blanket. (pause)

Cover yourself with a blanket if you like. (pause)

Do anything you need to do to become as comfortable as possible. (long pause for settling)

Set aside anything that's on your mind. You can always come back to the thoughts later if you like. Or you might find that some of the thoughts weren't so important, and you might choose to leave them aside for good. Either way, there's nothing you need to take care of right now.

Give your mind a chance to rest so you can come back to any thoughts with renewed clarity.

Set everything aside now for this time to rest and refresh. (long pause)

Take a deep breath in, and exhale, release.

Take another deep breath in and as you exhale, feel a sense of ease begin to set in.

Once again, deep breath in, and as you exhale, allow the peaceful feeling of ease to set in. (pause)

Scanning for tension now, check that shoulders are away from the ears. (pause)

Release the jaw.

Allow your head to sink into the support beneath it, or adjust if needed. (pause)

Scan your whole body, checking that you're as comfortable as can be. If not, make any adjustments needed or send messages of relaxation to any body parts where it's needed.

Send messages of relaxation to any body parts where it's needed. (long pause)

Begin to feel the stillness. Rest in that stillness. (pause)

Become aware of distant sounds. (long pause)

Allow your sense of hearing to extend out, receiving all sounds present at this moment, effortlessly and without analysis. Simply receiving with effortless awareness. (long pause)

Now bring your hearing into the room. Receiving sounds within the room. (long pause)

Listen for the soft sound of your body breathing. (long pause)

Feel the body resting. (long pause)

Be aware of your body breathing.

Your body breathing itself. (pause)

Nothing to do. (pause)

No need for concentration. Just effortless awareness. (pause)

Not thinking, just sensing.

Noticing.

Observing.

Effortless.

Pure awareness.

Effortless. (pause)

Yoga Nidra has now begun. (pause)

Sankalpa

Notice the sense of freedom in this effortless awareness. (pause)

This is the core of your being. Free and effortless.

Notice this natural freedom of your being. (pause)

You are free to move your awareness in any way you like, any time you like.

If ever you feel layers of heaviness or dullness upon this free, effortless awareness, know that beneath them is your true reality, your true being, which is ever free. (pause)

You can shift awareness freely, anytime you like.

Take a moment now, to picture yourself refreshed. Dullness, heaviness cast aside, refreshed. Refreshed in any way that feels good. (pause)

What does it look like? (long pause)

Sound like? (long pause)

Feel like? (long pause)

And now, if it feels right, planting this seed thought in this deeper aspect of your being, to help you effortlessly, spontaneously refresh:

"I am free. I refresh anytime I need." (pause)

"I am free. I refresh anytime I need." (pause)

"I am free. I refresh anytime I need." (pause)

Know this to be the seed of fresh new realities that will effortlessly spring forth from this moment on, whenever the need arises. (pause)

Rotation of Consciousness

Now taking a trip through the body, witnessing with curiosity and effortless awareness.

Allow the mind to hop from one body part to the next.

No need to think. Just awareness.

Awareness of any sensations, thoughts or feelings that might arise, but without attachment.

Simply noticing, and moving freely on.

Bring awareness to the point between the eyebrows

The point between the eyebrows

The hollow of the throat

The right shoulder

The right elbow

The middle of the right wrist

The right thumb

The tip of the index finger

Tip of the middle finger

Tip of the ring finger

Tip of the little finger

Back up to the right wrist

The elbow

The shoulder

The hollow of the throat

Sweeping awareness over to the left shoulder

The left elbow

The middle of the left wrist

The left thumb

Tip of the index finger

Tip of the middle finger

Tip of the ring finger

Tip of the little finger

Back up to the left wrist

The elbow

The shoulder

The hollow of the throat

The heart centre

The right side of the chest

The heart centre

The left side of the chest

The heart centre

The navel centre

The lower abdomen

The right hip joint

The right knee joint

The ankle joint

The right big toe

Tip of the second toe

Tip of the third toe

Tip of the fourth toe

Tip of the baby toe

Back up to the right ankle joint

Knee joint

Hip joint

Sweeping awareness to the left hip joint

Left knee joint

Ankle joint

The left big toe

Tip of the second toe

Tip of the third toe

Tip of the fourth toe

Tip of the baby toe

Back up to the left ankle

Knee joint

Hip joint

Lower abdomen

Navel centre (pause)

Heart centre (pause)

Hollow of the throat (pause)

The eyebrow centre

The eyebrow centre

The eyebrow centre (pause)

Breath Awareness

Now for a moment, bring awareness to the nostrils.

Without making any changes to the breath, feel that the breath is coming in from far away in two separate streams, through the nostrils. (pause)

Two streams coming in through the nostrils and meeting behind the point between the eyebrows, in the centre of the brain. (pause)

Keep breathing in this way, two streams from afar, meeting behind the point between the eyebrows, in the centre of the brain. (pause)

Breath coming in the right nostril stimulating activity, passion. (pause)

Breath coming in the left nostril stimulating stillness, rest. (pause)

Two streams coming in, for the perfect balance. (pause)

Two streams from afar, meeting behind the point between the eyebrows, in the centre of the brain. Keep breathing this way for the next several breaths. (pause for 30 seconds)

Opposites

Now beginning to manifest sensations in the body.

Start by developing the feeling of heaviness.

Each part of your body becoming heavier and heavier.

Feel the right leg heavy like stone, sinking, into the surface beneath you.

Left leg becoming heavier and heavier, sinking, into the surface beneath you.

Now feel heaviness in hips... back... chest... The whole torso, sinking into the surface beneath you.

Shoulders sinking. Arms and hands. Head. Heavy and sinking down into the surface beneath you.

Manifesting the sensation of heaviness in the whole body.

Entire body heavy, like stone. (pause)

Now, let go of the sensation of heaviness.

Completely let it go.

Release the sensation of heaviness from every part of the body.

Now awaken the sensation of lightness in the body.

Feel that every part of the body is filling up with lightness, like a helium balloon.

Body becoming lighter and lighter.

The right leg becoming light, lifting up.

Left leg filling up with lightness, floating up.

The right arm light. Left arm light.

The hips and torso, light as air.

And finally the head, filling with the sensation of lightness, floating right up.

Entire body, floating.

Experience lightness throughout the entire body. (pause)

Now, let go of the sensation of lightness.

Allow your body to gently release the feeling of floating.

Completely let go of the sensation of lightness.

Notice you can manifest or let go of the sensations of heaviness and lightness, any time you need. (pause)

You have the power to let go of the sensations of heaviness and lightness, any time you need. (pause)

Sankalpa

Now if you like, nourishing the seed thought for refreshment. If you repeat it with feeling and awareness, it will not fail. Say to yourself mentally,

"I am free. I refresh anytime I need." (pause)

"I am free. I refresh anytime I need." (pause)

"I am free. I refresh anytime I need." (pause)

Know that fresh new realities are already beginning to effortlessly spring forth. (pause)

Take a moment to visualize, and *feel*, the joy of your refreshment already manifested. (long pause)

Externalization

Become aware of your breath.

Your body resting, breathing itself. (pause)

Listen for the soft sound of your body breathing. (long pause)

Feel the sensation of your body breathing. (long pause)

Allow awareness to rise back to the surface. Back to the body and the space you're in.

Be aware of sounds in the room. (long pause)

Visualize yourself resting peacefully in the room. (long pause)

Know that the practice is coming to an end.

Take a deep breath in, feel awareness rising even more, back into the body.

Yoga Nidra is now complete. (pause)

Beginning gentle movements, wiggle your fingers, wiggle your toes. (pause)

Make any larger movements – move your feet, legs, hands, arms, whatever you like, however you like, and if you're lying down, when you're ready, roll to the right side. (long pause)

Take a few deep breaths, reminding yourself to take notice – after this reset, you might find yourself naturally, spontaneously, making new choices, starting new habits, letting go of heaviness, manifesting lightness. (pause)

Make a note to observe any shifts in feeling refreshed and free to shift anytime you like. (long pause)

And now, if you were lying down, keeping your eyes closed if you can, slowly press yourself up to sitting. (long pause)

Say to yourself mentally one more time: "I am free. I refresh anytime I need." (long pause)

We'll finish by chanting Om and Shanti, three times each.

Take a deep breath in.

Om Om Om Shanti Shanti Shanti (pause)

Before opening your eyes, take one more moment to remember your joyful vision of your fresh start. And when you're ready, softly open your eyes with a fresh new perspective.

Pure Abundance *(25 min.)*

A practice to help you open up to pure abundance.

Suggested Pre- and Post-Practices:

- Consider beginning with an asana practice or a few minutes of simple stretches to release bodily tension – such as seated or standing shoulder rolls, twists, side bends and forward folds.
- Prepare with a few minutes of Yoni Mudra for increased receptivity and improved intuition.
- Prepare with the mantra of Om for connection to the higher Self.

Settling

Getting comfortable, lying down or sitting, supported.

Choosing any position that's comfortable right now. Getting ready for this practice for opening to abundance.

Tuck something under your head for support if it feels good.

Cover yourself with a blanket if you like.

Make any choices you need to get as comfortable as possible. (long pause for settling)

Check for any potential distractions. Maybe a wrinkle in your blanket, a crooked pillow – anything that might distract you from your practice.

If you find anything, adjust it now. (long pause)

Now bring awareness to your feet.

Send a comforting message to your feet to relax or simply send a feeling of ease. You can do this in any way that feels good to you.

Sending awareness to the feet to release into ease, comfort, relaxation. (pause)

And now sending a message or feeling to the legs to release into ease, comfort, relaxation. (pause) And now the hips… back… arms… shoulders… jaw… forehead.

Scan your whole body, making sure you're as comfortable as can be. If not, adjust in any way you need. (pause)

Feel yourself settling in. (pause)

Take a deep breath in… and as you exhale, let go of any need to *do*. Right now, you are just *being*.

Resting, effortlessly.

In the comfort you've created.

Not thinking. *Feeling*.

Body is relaxed.

Awareness continues on.

Effortless.

Yoga Nidra has now begun. (pause)

Sankalpa

Now, with the intention to connect with the quality of abundance, take a moment to picture yourself living an abundant life. (pause)

Visualize yourself living in abundance. In as much detail as you can. (long pause)

Feel yourself experiencing that abundance. (long pause)

And if it feels right, repeat mentally, with *joy*: "I am abundant", three times. (long pause)

Know that this seed thought has been planted, and has already begun manifesting.

Rotation of Consciousness

Now moving awareness through the body.

Awareness moving from point to point, effortlessly.

Awareness of any sensations or thoughts that might arise, but remaining unattached.

Start with awareness of the point between the eyebrows

Effortless awareness of the point between the eyebrows

The hollow of the throat

The right shoulder joint

Passive awareness

The right elbow joint

Wrist joint

The right thumb

Tip of the index finger

Tip of the middle finger

Tip of the ring finger

Tip of the little finger

Effortless awareness

The right wrist joint

Elbow joint

Shoulder joint

Hollow of the throat

Shifting to the left shoulder joint

Elbow joint

Wrist joint

The left thumb

Tip of the index finger

Tip of the middle finger

Tip of the ring finger

Tip of the little finger

Not thinking. Feeling.

Effortless.

The left wrist joint

Elbow joint

Shoulder joint

Hollow of the throat

The heart centre

The right side of the chest

The heart centre

The left side of the chest

The heart centre

The heart centre

The heart centre

Resting awareness at the heart centre. Not thinking. Feeling. (pause)

Breath Awareness

Now become aware of the breath at the heart centre. (pause)

Notice on the inhalation, expansion.

As you exhale, contraction.

Watch the natural breath.

Simply be aware.

Inhale, expansion.

Exhale, contraction.

Expansion.

Contraction.

Follow this movement for a several breaths now. Expansion, contraction. (pause for 30 seconds)

Opposites

Now manifesting opposite sensations in the body. First, beginning to manifest the sensation *opposite* to abundance, the sensation of *lack*. If it feels safe, imagine just for a moment that you lost something important to you – a job, money, a relationship. Try to imagine it clearly and notice the sensation. Is it a sensation of contraction or expansion? Notice the heart centre – does it feel more closed or open? (pause)

This is the sensation of lack.

Now let go of the sensation of lack.

Completely let it go.

Release the sensation of lack *entirely*. (pause)

Realize that you have just *created* the sensation of lack and *released* the sensation of lack, using only your mind. Recognize the power of the mind to *create* the sensation of lack and *let go* of the sensation of lack. (pause)

Now manifesting the sensation of abundance.

If it feels good, imagine for a moment that you gained something fulfilling – a job, money, a relationship, or anything else. Try to picture it vividly and notice the sensation. Is it a sensation of contraction or expansion? Notice the heart centre – does it feel more closed or open? (long pause)

This is the sensation of abundance. (pause)

Now let go of the sensation of abundance.

Completely let it go.

Realize that you have just *released* the sensation of abundance and *created* the sensation of abundance, using only your mind. Recognize the power of the mind to *let go* of the sensation of abundance and *create* the sensation of abundance. (pause)

Now noticing for a moment...

Recall again the thing that gave the sensation of abundance. (long pause)

Notice the sensation of expansion. (pause)

Now imagine it was lost. (pause)

Notice the sense of contraction again. (pause)

Gain and loss. An inseparable pair of opposites, sometimes out of your control. But what *is* in your control is where your awareness lies.

Look within for a moment.

Shifting from thinking to feeling again.

Be aware within.

Awareness of your ever-free soul.

Pure awareness.

Ever free from the pairs of opposites.

Ever free from *any* external factors.

An endless abundance of potential, freedom and ever-lasting peace.

You, the soul, are truly abundant.

Infinitely abundant.

Unlimited.

Constant.

Eternally. (pause)

With confidence, know that all abundance *already* resides within you.

All abundance *already* resides within you. (pause)

Notice your heart expand.

Take a moment to feel the sensation of an expanded, open heart. (pause)

Open to receive. The more open, the more you can receive. (pause)

Receiving abundance – job, money, relationships or anything else, but *without attachment*. Understand that fear, fear of loss, contracts the heart. (pause)

Fear closes the heart from receiving.

Stay open.

Openness comes from knowing you're already full. Already infinitely abundant. Lacking nothing. (pause)

Feel the expansion.

You are *already* abundant.

Heart open to receive, with ease, intelligence and healthy boundaries for wellbeing.

Heart open to receive, with ease, intelligence and healthy boundaries for wellbeing.

Awareness of the heart centre, opening, expanding.

Awareness of the heart centre, opening, expanding. (pause)

If you *feel* abundant, the heart is expanded, open to receive more.

If you simply *hope* for abundance, it means the feeling of lack is still present, heart is closed and not open to receive.

So now, take a moment to *feel* that you already are abundant, as vividly as you can.

Feeling abundant, heart open to receive.

Feeling abundant, heart open to receive.

(long pause)

Sankalpa

Now if you like, mentally repeat "I am abundant", three times again, with full feeling. (long pause)

Know that this thought has been recorded in your being and is already changing the course of your life.

Externalization

Bring awareness back to your heart centre. (pause)

Notice the heart centre rising on inhalation, falling on exhalation. (pause)

Bring awareness back to your body.

Yoga Nidra is now complete. (pause)

Feel your body peacefully resting. (pause)

Feel the support beneath you. (pause)

Notice the temperature of the space you're in. (pause)

Notice the sounds. Close sounds, far sounds. (long pause)

Take a few deep breaths. (long pause)

Now wiggle your fingers and toes.

Stretch or move your body, any way you like. (pause)

If you're lying down, when you're ready, roll to your right side. Take a few deep breaths here. And if it feels good, mentally repeat once more, "I am abundant". (long pause)

If you were lying down, keeping your eyes closed, slowly press yourself up to sitting. (long pause)

We'll finish by chanting Om three times and Shanti three times. We'll pause for silence, and when you're ready, open your eyes.

Take a deep breath in…

Om Om Om Shanti Shanti Shanti (pause)

Enjoy the sensation of abundance throughout your day.

Tranquility & Ease (Pitta Pacifying) *(25 min.)*

A practice that can be used by anyone to inspire a sense of tranquility and ease, but is particularly beneficial for people with abundant Pitta dosha.

Suggested Pre- and Post-Practices:

- Begin with a few wide-legged, gentle sun salutations to release tension, followed by grounding, wide-legged poses. Avoid heat-producing asanas, pranayama or other practices.

- You might also begin with a short Prana Restorative Yoga practice, that has a balance of stimulation and relaxation. (See my Prana Restorative Yoga course at tamaraskyhawk.com for details.)

- Prepare or finish with a few minutes of holding Anjali Mudra, to move awareness from the head to the heart and inspire humility.

- Consider beginning with Sitali pranayama (breathing), for cooling.

- Prepare or finish with this Shanti Mantra, to stimulate compassion for others.

    Sarvesham svastir bhavatu

    Sarvesham shantir bhavatu

    Sarvesham purnam bhavatu

    Sarvesham mangalam bhavatu

(May prosperity be unto all, may peace be unto all, may fullness be unto all, may auspiciousness be unto all)

Settling

Choose your most comfortable position. You know best what that is. Maybe lying in savasana, or sitting up, supported. (pause)

Getting ready for this Yoga Nidra practice to inspire a sense of tranquility and ease. Tranquility and ease that is well deserved. (pause)

Set yourself up with your favourite head support, bolster under your knees if you enjoy that. Eye pillow or scarf if it's soothing. Taking your time to get your set-up just the way you like it. (long pause for settling)

If you're lying in savasana, legs and arms are away from the body. (pause)

In any position, shoulders are away from the ears to create a sense of ease and openness. (pause)

Taking care to make any adjustments needed, knowing it will help you make the most of your practice. A comfortable set-up is the foundation of your Yoga Nidra practice.

Pull out all the stops. Treat yourself to the most comfortable set-up possible.

This is your time to simply rest.

You've definitely earned it. (pause)

If you feel it's helpful, make a mental note to set aside anything that's on your mind. You can always come back to things later if you like.

Right now, there's nothing you need to do. Set everything aside for this time to rest. (long pause)

Take a deep breath in… and as you exhale, feel that you let go of any urge to do. Letting go of any urge to do anything.

Deep breath in… and once again, exhale, letting go of any urge to do.

You've already done so much.

For all you do, you deserve time to rest.

Just rest.

You might begin to notice your body relaxing, softening, chilling out.

Be aware of any sensations of relaxing, softening, chilling out. (pause)

Now beginning the process of becoming aware of the senses, then letting them rest, too.

Become aware of any scent in the room.

Take deep breaths, noticing any scent in the room. (long pause)

And now, noticing scents closer to you. The scent of your clothing… your hair… the scent within your nostrils. (long pause)

Now allow your sense of smell to rest. Moving awareness on to visualization.

Picture the room you're in. The ceiling… the walls… anything in the room… the floor… the space directly around you… visualizing. (long pause)

Now allow your sense of sight to rest.

Feel the texture of the props you're using. Soft, hard. (pause)

Feel the texture of your clothing – smooth, rough. (long pause)

Now allow your sense of touch to rest.

Be aware of sounds. Become aware of sounds far away. (long pause)

Now be aware of sounds closer in, within the room. (long pause)

Be aware of the closest sound, the sound of your body breathing. (long pause)

Be aware of your body breathing.

Your body breathing itself. (pause)

Nothing to do.

No need for concentration.

Just effortless awareness.

Feel all experience slowing down.

All experience becoming more and more tranquil.

Still.

Tranquil.

Effortless. (pause)

Yoga Nidra has now begun. (pause)

Sankalpa

If you have a sankalpa, allow it to arise in your awareness now. If you don't have a sankalpa, you can use the affirmation: "I am at ease", or any other statement that feels good. (long pause)

Allow the *feeling* of your sankalpa to grow. Feel it refreshing your soul, like a tall, cool drink of water. (long pause)

With confidence, repeat your sankalpa, or "I am at ease", three times mentally now. (long pause)

You can be certain your sankalpa is already working its magic from deep within you. Manifesting your heart's desire, bringing a sense of ease to your heart. (pause)

Rotation of Consciousness

Moving awareness into the body.

Moving awareness from point to point.

Begin with awareness of the point between the eyebrows

Nothing you need to think about or do, simply be aware

Effortless awareness of the point between the eyebrows

The hollow of the throat

The right shoulder joint

The right elbow joint

The right wrist joint

The right thumb
Tip of the index finger
Tip of the middle finger
Tip of the ring finger
Tip of the little finger
Back up to the wrist joint
Elbow joint
Shoulder joint
Hollow of the throat
Shifting to the left shoulder joint
Left elbow joint
Left wrist joint
The left thumb
Tip of the index finger
Tip of the middle finger
Tip of the ring finger
Tip of the little finger
Back up to the wrist joint
Elbow joint
Shoulder joint
Hollow of the throat
The heart centre (pause)
The hollow of the throat (pause)
The point between the eyebrows (pause)
The tip of the nose
Resting awareness at the tip of the nose (pause)

Breath Awareness

Become aware of the breath.

The breath in the nostrils. (pause)

No need to change the breath in any way.

Simply watching the breath.

Notice on the inhalation, cool air coming in through the nostrils.

Cool air, streaming in through the nostrils with each inhalation.

Contraction of the nostrils, and cool air streaming in. (long pause)

Move awareness to just the left nostril.

Feel cool air coming in through the left nostril, with each inhalation. (long pause)

Now follow an inhalation through the left nostril and as you exhale, feel that you exhale through the right nostril.

Inhale cool air through the left nostril, exhale warm air from the right nostril.

Cool air streaming in the left, warm air going out the right.

Cooling the body through the breath.

Cool air in the left nostril, warm air out the right.

If it feels relaxed and easy, keep watching the breath in this way. Or if you prefer, simply focus on the left nostril. (long pause)

Symbols/Visualization

Now accessing the subconscious mind, with symbols to stimulate a sense of tranquility, ease, rest.

There's nothing you need to do.

Symbols will be mentioned.

Simply be aware of anything that arises, either from memory or imagination.

Watching, with detached awareness. (pause)

A soaring eagle (repeat 3 times)

An ice rink (repeat 3 times)

A lounge chair (repeat 3 times)

A glowing full moon (repeat 3 times)

A field of lavender (repeat 3 times)

Fog on a still lake (repeat 3 times)

(pause)

Sankalpa

And now, if you have a sankalpa, allow it to arise in your awareness. If you don't have a sankalpa, you can use: "I am at ease", or the statement you chose earlier. (pause)

Allow the *feeling* of your sankalpa to grow. Feel it refreshing your soul, like a tall, cool drink of water. (long pause)

With confidence, repeat your sankalpa, or "I am at ease", three times mentally now. (long pause)

You can be certain your sankalpa is already working its magic from deep within you. Manifesting your heart's desire. (pause)

There's nothing else you need to do.

You can feel at ease knowing your sankalpa is already manifesting.

Take a minute now to dive into that sense of ease and peace.

Ease and peace at the heart centre.

Rest your awareness at the heart centre for the next minute. (pause for 1 minute)

Externalization

If your mind wandered, become aware of your heart centre.

Awareness of the heart centre.

Feel your body breathing. (pause)

Feel your chest rising and falling.

Feel the weight of any clothing on the chest. (long pause)

Notice the texture of any props you're using or clothing you're wearing. (long pause)

Picture the room you're in. The space around you... the floor... the walls... the ceiling. (long pause)

Know that your Yoga Nidra practice is wrapping up.

Take a couple of deep breaths and notice any scent in the room.

Take deep breaths, noticing any scent in the room. (long pause)

Yoga Nidra is now complete. (pause)

Move your body in any way that feels good. Stretch, roll your ankles and wrists. Maybe draw your knees into your chest if you're lying down. Whatever feels nice. (long pause)

And if you're lying down, when you're ready, roll to the right side. (pause)

Take a few deep breaths, awareness coming back into your day, holding any sensation of ease, tranquility or rest from your practice today. (long pause)

Now taking your time, if you were lying down, move slowly up to sitting.

There's no rush. (long pause)

Sitting with comfort and ease, take a deep breath in... and a long breath out.

If you like, mentally repeat your sankalpa or "I am at ease", one more time, to keep it top of mind. (pause)

We'll finish by chanting Om and Shanti, three times each.

Take a deep breath in.

Om Om Om Shanti Shanti Shanti (pause)

When you're ready, slowly open your eyes.

Steadiness & Support (Vata Pacifying) (25-30 min.)

A practice that can be used by anyone to inspire a sense of stability, but is particularly beneficial for people with abundant Vata dosha.

Suggested Pre- and Post-Practices:

- Consider beginning with restorative yoga poses, seated poses and movements, child's pose, squatting.
- Prepare with a few minutes of chanting the universal mantra, Om, to calm and soothe.
- Prepare with Nadi Shodhana pranayama (breathing), to calm and balance the mind.
- Prepare or finish with meditation using a grounding mudra, such as Prithvi Mudra, the mudra of the earth element.
- Begin and/or finish with self-massage on the shoulders, lower back, legs, then feet.

Settling

Snuggle up in your favourite resting position – on your back, your side, your abdomen, or sitting, supported.

Any position that feels supportive is just right.

Getting ready for your Yoga Nidra practice for nourishment and steadiness. (pause)

Get as cozy and warm as you like. The cozier the better. Give yourself all the things – something soft and supportive under your head, warm socks, sweater, blankets, bolsters, cushions… whatever you need. Take your time to get it just right. This is your special time for self care. (long pause for settling)

And now, once you're all tucked in, safe and snuggled up, take a moment to ask yourself, "Is there anything else I could do to feel more cozy?" (long pause)

If anything came to you, make the upgrade now. Upgrading to decadent coziness. Or if you're already there, begin to let go into that beautiful support and comfort. (long pause)

Now that you're perfectly cocooned, and supported by the solid ground beneath you, if it feels good, you can surrender to gravity.

Begin to feel your shoulders relax… neck relax… arms and hands relax… back relax… hips… legs… feet.

Whole body, letting go into the steady support. Feel the support, steady, like a rock.

Know that you can move anytime you like, but if it feels good to just be held here in this steady support for a while, then enjoy that non-doing. (pause)

Body is resting.

Now beginning the process of becoming aware of the senses, then letting them rest, too.

Become aware of any scent in the room.

Take deep breaths, noticing any scent in the room. (long pause)

And now, scents closer to you. The scent of your clothing… your hair… the scent within your nostrils. (long pause)

Now allow your sense of smell to rest.

Moving awareness on to visualization.

Picture the room you're in. The ceiling… the walls… anything in the room… the floor… the space directly around you… visualizing. (long pause)

Now allow your sense of sight to rest.

Feel the texture of the props you're using. Soft, hard. (pause)

Feel the texture of your clothing – smooth, rough. (long pause)

Now allow your sense of touch to rest.

Be aware of sounds. Become aware of sounds far away. (long pause)

Now be aware of sounds closer in, within the room. (long pause)

Be aware of the closest sound, the sound of your body breathing. (long pause)

Yoga Nidra has now begun. (pause)

Sankalpa

If you have a sankalpa, allow it to arise in your awareness now. If you don't have a sankalpa, you can use the affirmation: "I am supported", or any other statement that feels good. (long pause)

Allow the *feeling* of your sankalpa to grow. Feel it nourishing your soul, bringing warmth to your heart, like a warm cup of tea. (long pause)

With a sure sense of steady confidence, repeat your sankalpa or "I am supported", three times mentally now. (long pause)

You can be certain your sankalpa is already working its magic from deep within you. Bringing your heart's desire to life and a sense of peace to your heart. (pause)

Rotation of Consciousness

Moving awareness into the body.

Moving awareness from point to point.

Begin with awareness of the right side of the body

Be aware of the right hand

Right hand thumb

Index finger

Middle finger

Ring finger

Little finger
Palm of the hand
Back of the hand
Right wrist
Right lower arm
Right elbow
Right upper arm
Right shoulder
Moving over to the left side of the body
Be aware of the left hand
Left hand thumb
Index finger
Middle finger
Ring finger
Little finger
Palm of the hand
Back of the hand
Left wrist
Left lower arm
Left elbow
Left upper arm
Left shoulder
Steady awareness
Moving up to the crown of the head
Crown of the head
Forehead
Right temple
Left temple
Right eyebrow

Left eyebrow

Eyebrow centre

Right eye

Left eye

Right ear

Left ear

Right cheek

Left cheek

Right nostril

Left nostril

Upper lip

Lower lip

Chin

Throat centre

Right collarbone

Left collarbone

Right side of the chest

Left side of the chest

Heart centre

Navel

Lower abdomen

Move awareness back up to the crown of the head

Back of the head

Back of the neck

Right shoulder blade

Left shoulder blade

Upper back

Middle back

Lower back

Sacrum

Right hip

Right thigh

Right knee

Right lower leg

Right ankle

Right heel

Sole of the foot

Top of the foot

Right big toe

Second toe

Third toe

Fourth toe

Fifth toe

Steady awareness

Move over to the left hip

Left thigh

Left knee

Left lower leg

Left ankle

Left heel

Sole of the foot

Top of the foot

Left big toe

Second toe

Third toe

Fourth toe

Fifth toe

Be aware of the whole right side of the body (pause)

The whole left side of the body (pause)

The whole body together

The whole body together

The whole body together (long pause)

Breath Awareness

Now become aware of the navel.

Notice the body breathing itself. Just noticing.

Abdomen gently rises and falls with each breath.

Nothing for you to do.

Simply witnessing.

Awake and aware.

Be aware of the navel.

The navel centre is your centre for digestive fire, and creating warmth in the body.

Feel that with each breath in, you're pulling energy down to the navel centre. (pause)

Each breath in, pulling energy down to the navel centre.

The navel centre transforms the energy into heat, and it's radiated out to the whole body. Warmth radiated out to the whole body. (pause)

Visualize a blazing fire in the belly. Blazing fire at the navel centre. Flames fanned bigger with every in-breath. (long pause)

Feel that with each inhale, the fire at the navel centre grows stronger.

With each exhale, heat moves out to all parts of the body. Right out to the fingers, toes and beyond. (pause)

Inhale fuelling the fire.

Exhale the warmth spreads.

Inhale fuelling the fire.

Exhale the warmth spreads.

Keep breathing this way for the next minute, feeling heat created in the body. (pause for 1 minute)

Symbols/Visualization

Now accessing the subconscious mind with symbols that are grounding, steadying, comforting.

There's nothing you need to do.

Symbols will be mentioned.

Simply be aware of anything that arises, either from memory or imagination.

Watching, with detached awareness. (pause)

Sand dunes (repeat 3 times)

A hippopotamus (repeat 3 times)

Water evaporating on a hot rock (repeat 3 times)

Sunglasses (repeat 3 times)

Stonehenge (repeat 3 times)

A steaming bowl of sticky rice (repeat 3 times)

Sunbeam on a carpet (repeat 3 times)

A thick, oversized beach towel (repeat 3 times)

A hot bath (pause)

Sankalpa

And now, if you have a sankalpa, allow it to arise in your awareness. If you don't have a sankalpa, you can use: "I am supported", or the statement you chose earlier. (pause)

Allow the *feeling* of your sankalpa to grow. Feel it nourishing your soul again, bringing its same warmth to your heart, like a warm cup of tea. (long pause)

With a sure sense of steady confidence, repeat your sankalpa three times mentally now. (long pause)

Your sankalpa has been planted, with deep, strong roots in your being.

There's nothing else you need to do.

You can feel comforted knowing your sankalpa is supporting you from deep within.

Take a minute now to dive into that peace and comfort.

Peace and comfort at the heart centre.

Rest your awareness at the heart centre. (pause for 1-5 minutes)

Externalization

If your mind wandered, become aware of your heart centre.

Awareness of the heart centre.

Feel your body breathing. (pause)

Feel your chest rising and falling.

Feel the weight of any clothing or blankets on the chest. (long pause)

Notice the texture of any props you're using or clothing you're wearing. (long pause)

Picture the room you're in. The space around you... the floor... the walls... the ceiling. (long pause)

Know that your Yoga Nidra practice is wrapping up.

Take a couple of deep breaths and notice any scent in the room.

Take deep breaths, noticing any scent in the room. (long pause)

Yoga Nidra is now complete. (pause)

Move your body in any way that feels good. Stretch, roll your ankles and wrists. If you're lying down, maybe hug your knees into your chest. Rock around on your back. Whatever feels nice. (long pause)

Now also if you're lying down, when you're ready, roll to your right side. (pause)

Take a few deep breaths, awareness coming back into your day, holding any sensation of steadiness, support, comfort or warmth from your practice today. (long pause)

Now taking your time, if you were lying down, move slowly up to sitting.

There's no rush. (long pause)

Sitting with comfort and steadiness, take a deep breath in... and a long breath out.

If you like, mentally repeat your sankalpa or "I am supported", one more time, to keep it top of mind. (long pause)

We'll finish by chanting Om and Shanti, three times each.

Take a deep breath in.

Om Om Om Shanti Shanti Shanti (pause)

When you're ready, slowly open your eyes.

Peaceful Orchard *(25-30 min.)*

Take an excursion to a lush, peaceful orchard and receive the gifts it has to offer you.

Suggested Pre- and Post-Practices:

- Begin with a relaxed asana or movement practice that loosens up the joints and major muscles.
- Begin or finish with a few minutes of holding Anjali Mudra to inspire feelings of humility and connection.
- Prepare or finish with a Shanti Mantra such as:

    Sarvesham svastir bhavatu

    Sarvesham shantir bhavatu

    Sarvesham purnam bhavatu

    Sarvesham mangalam bhavatu

    (May prosperity be unto all, may peace be unto all, may fullness be unto all, may auspiciousness be unto all)

Settling

Prepare yourself a comfortable spot for a peaceful Yoga Nidra journey to a beautiful orchard.

Setting up in any way that resonates with you today. Lying down in any way you like, sitting supported or reclined… whatever is resonating today for this peaceful journey you're about to embark on. (pause)

In any case, you'll want to be sure your head is supported with something soft, and you'll want to do your best to reduce tension or irritation that might distract you from your practice. Loosening clothing, removing jewellery, smoothing any blankets beneath you or on top of you. Removing any potential distractions. Taking time to create your perfect set-up. (long pause for settling)

And now, begin to release tension from the body. Allow your forehead and jaw to soften… neck and shoulders soften… arms and hands soften… back softening… legs softening. Whole body, softening. Releasing tension.

Feel your body begin to relax. (pause)

Body resting, peacefully and still. You can move anytime you like, but if this stillness feels sweet, carry on.

Bringing awareness to the senses, one by one, then letting them rest.

Start with awareness of any scent.

Take deep breaths, noticing any scent. (long pause)

Maybe you noticed some scent, maybe not. Both are fine. Simply noticing.

Now allow your sense of smell to rest. Moving on to sight.

With eyes still closed, see the outside of the building you're in. (long pause)

Now bring awareness closer, see the farthest wall of the room you're in. (long pause)

Now see your body, resting in the room. (long pause)

Allow the sense of sight to rest now.

Bring awareness to any sounds outside the building or outside the room. (long pause)

Maybe you notice some sounds, maybe not. Both are fine. Simply being aware. Detached awareness.

Now listening for the sound of your breath. (long pause)

Maybe you hear it, maybe not. It doesn't matter. Simply being aware, effortlessly.

Allow your awareness to be effortless. (pause)

Body is resting, external senses are resting.

Beginning a journey of awareness.

There's nothing you need to do.

Effortless awareness. (pause)

Yoga Nidra has now begun. (pause)

Rotation of Consciousness

While your body rests comfortably, allow your awareness to travel on, taking a journey to a peaceful, lush orchard. (pause)

A sunny, lush orchard. All your own. Completely private. Miles and miles of rolling hills surrounding you. (pause)

In this orchard, there are trees of many types, some with fragrant blooms. Some with juicy, ripe, fragrant fruits in vibrant colours. Apple, peach, cherry, pear... (long pause)

In this fragrant, peaceful orchard, with no one around but you and the singing birds, happily feasting on the fruits, find a soft, grassy spot to lay down a picnic blanket. (long pause)

Now laying your picnic blanket down, smooth it out and lie down comfortably for some relaxation. (long pause)

Lying in the warm air, shaded by the trees, sunshine all around.

Lying on your picnic blanket, getting ready to practice your Yoga Nidra rotation of consciousness.

Lulling yourself into relaxation.

Moving awareness within the body.

Beginning with effortless awareness of the point between your eyebrows

Effortless awareness of the point between your eyebrows

Maybe noticing the sun's light here (pause)

Move awareness to the hollow of the throat

Moving freely to the right shoulder joint

Elbow joint

Wrist joint

The right thumb

The tip of the index finger

Tip of the middle finger

Tip of the ring finger

Tip of the little finger

The right wrist joint

Elbow joint

Shoulder joint

Hollow of the throat

Over to the left shoulder joint

Elbow joint

Wrist joint

The left thumb

Tip of the index finger

Tip of the middle finger

Tip of the ring finger

Tip of the little finger

Back up to the left wrist joint

Elbow joint

Shoulder joint

Hollow of the throat

The heart centre

The right side of the chest

The heart centre

The left side of the chest

The heart centre

The heart centre

The heart centre

Noticing the sun's warmth at the heart centre (long pause)

Breath Awareness

Expanding awareness to the whole body now.

Feel the sun's warmth and energy permeating your whole body. (long pause)

Noticing the gentle wave of your natural breath. (long pause)

Noticing that with each effortless inhale, you draw in fresh air and energy. (pause)

Every effortless inhale, drawing in fresh air and energy. (pause)

As you exhale, you release a gift for the trees in the orchard. Carbon dioxide. The trees happily breathe in this carbon dioxide. (pause)

And in exchange, the trees breathe out oxygen, a gift to you. (pause)

Noticing this perfect, beautiful exchange.

Effortlessly, you breathe in the gift from the trees – energizing oxygen.

And effortlessly as you exhale, you give energy to the trees.

Breathing in energy.

Breathing out energy.

Effortless. (pause)

Breathing in, receiving.

Breathing out, giving.

Effortless. (pause)

Continue to be aware of this perfect, effortless, Divine exchange between you and the trees in the orchard, for the next minute. (pause 1 minute)

Symbols/Visualization

Now with the body and energy at peace, get ready to explore this beautiful orchard.

Notice the vibrant colours of the fruits. Juicy red apples... crimson cherries... pastel peaches... yellow pears.

One of these fruit trees is particularly intriguing you, so you get up from your picnic blanket and walk over to that fruit tree. (pause)

Closer now, you can see there's an abundance of fruit. Search for a ripe, juicy one. (pause)

Pick the piece of fruit and hold it in your hand. Feel its shape and texture. (pause) Notice its warmth.

Take a bite if you like, notice the flavour, the sweetness, the juiciness. (long pause)

A cute little bird lands close by, on a branch in the tree. (pause)

She's very interested in your fruit.

If you like, hold out your hand and she'll come to you, to peck at the fruit. (long pause)

Take a moment to appreciate the harmony here in the orchard. Your private, beautiful orchard. (long pause)

And now, return back to your picnic blanket. Lie down comfortably, hands over your heart in gratitude for this beautiful experience. (long pause)

As you lie down comfortably, allow awareness to move deep into your heart centre. (pause)

Heart full, from your sweet experience in the orchard. (pause)

In this peace, there is clarity and connection.

Your connection is ripe to receive guidance.

If you'd like to ask for any guidance, you'll have several minutes to receive it now or simply allow awareness to enjoy the peace in any way you'd like. (pause for 2-6 minutes)

Externalization

Bringing awareness back to the heart centre, prepare to say goodbye to the orchard. Know you can come back here again, anytime you like. Everything you need is within you. (long pause)

Saying goodbye to the orchard now. Thankful for any positive experiences you had here. (long pause)

Awareness travelling back to the body now.

Back to the heart centre of your physical body.

Notice the gentle wave of the chest rising and falling with each breath. (pause)

Gentle wave of breath, rising and falling.

Picture your body, resting in the room. (pause)

Take a couple of deep breaths in, noticing any scent in the room. (long pause)

External senses reactivating.

Awareness back in the body.

Yoga Nidra is now complete. (pause)

Taking a few deep breaths now and notice sensation coming back to the body, even more. (long pause)

Wiggle your fingers and toes and feel the sweet little sparks of energy. (pause)

Stretch or move your body. Move freely and with care. (long pause)

And if you're lying down, when you're ready, roll to your right side.

Take a few deep breaths. (long pause)

Remember your experience in the beautiful orchard. What would you like to take with you from your experience today? Were there any insights, positive feelings or guidance you'd like to bring to the surface of your awareness? (long pause)

If you were lying down, press yourself gently up to sitting.

Keep your eyes closed if you can.

Take as much time as you need. (long pause)

Sitting up, back as straight as you can make it, top of the head rising toward the ceiling.

Take a few deep breaths in, feeling the energy rising. (pause for 3 breaths)

We'll finish by chanting Om and Shanti three times each.

Feel the energy revitalize and awaken you as you chant.

Take a deep breath in.

Om Om Om Shanti Shanti Shanti (pause)

And welcome back.

Vibrancy Rising *(25-35 min.)*

Allow vibrancy to rise to the surface and shine through body and mind.

Suggested Pre- and Post-Practices:

- Consider beginning with a minute or two of simple rotations for the joints, done standing or sitting – neck, shoulders, wrists, back, hips, knees, ankles.

- Consider finishing with a quick self-massage of neck, shoulders, scalp, hands, arms, lower back, abdomen, legs, feet.

- Begin with Kapalabhati pranayama (breathing), to stimulate energy.

- Begin or finish with meditation using Bhairavi Mudra, stimulating Shakti and manifestation.

Settling

Getting cozy, lying down or sitting, supported, whatever feels right for you, right now. Getting ready for this practice to awaken your vibrancy.

Tuck a thin pillow or folded blanket under your head if you like.

Cover yourself with a blanket if you like.

Do anything you need to do to get as comfy as possible. (long pause for settling)

Doing a check in now to notice if there's anything that might distract you – a tight waistband, cold hands, an uncomfortable fold or twist in your clothing – anything that might distract you.

Make any adjustments you need, now. (long pause)

Now beginning the process of melting tension. Starting at your feet, allow your feet to let go of any tension, melting.

Now the legs, tension melting.

The hips… (pause)

The whole back, melting in to the surface supporting you. (pause)

Arms melt… shoulders melt… neck… jaw… forehead and scalp.

Notice the sensation of stillness settling in.

The opportunity to simply rest.

Nothing asked of you.

Nothing to accomplish.

Simply being.

Take a deep breath in… and as you exhale, settle further into this sensation of simply being. (pause)

All the cares of the day fall to the side.

You can release them in this moment. (pause)

Allow your mental "to-do" list to fall to the side. You can come back to any important thoughts after your practice, but for now, set them aside.

Or, if there are thoughts you'd like to let go of entirely, feel free to let go of them entirely. (long pause)

In this moment, let everything fall to the side, giving you space to freely dive within, connect with your self and allow your natural vibrancy to shine forth.

This journey to reconnect with your natural vibrancy will be effortless.

The more effortless your awareness, the more easily your vibrancy will shine through. (pause)

Effortless.

Radiant. (pause)

Yoga Nidra has now begun. (pause)

Sankalpa

Now, if you have a sankalpa that fills you with joy, allow it to arise in your awareness.

If not, if it feels good you can use the affirmation: "I am vibrant". Or simply hold the feeling or a memory of vibrancy. (pause)

If it feels good, repeat your sankalpa or "I am vibrant" now. (pause)

Know that it is manifesting the instant you repeat the thought.

If it feels good, repeat it once more, feeling that it is manifesting even further now, with more strength. (pause)

And finally, if you like, repeat it one more time, feeling that as you do, your sankalpa is manifesting with great strength, ease and speed. (pause)

Take a moment now to feel the joy of your sankalpa already becoming reality. (long pause)

Rotation of Consciousness

Now beginning to enliven the whole body with energy.

It's very effortless.

Where awareness goes, energy flows.

Simply shift awareness freely from point to point, and energy will *automatically* be swept throughout your entire body.

Begin with awareness of the right hand

Right hand thumb

Index finger

Middle finger

Ring finger

Little finger

Sweeping awareness over to the left hand thumb

Index finger

Middle finger

Ring finger

Little finger

Energizing the body, effortlessly, simply by moving awareness

Move awareness over to the right wrist

Left wrist

Right elbow

Left elbow

Right shoulder

Left shoulder

Hollow of the throat

Sweeping awareness to the back of the head near the top

Crown of the head

Eyebrow centre

Right eyebrow

Left eyebrow

Right eye

Left eye

Right ear

Left ear

Right cheek

Left cheek

Tip of the nose

Upper lip

Lower lip

Chin

Hollow of the throat

Heart centre

Right side of the chest

Heart centre

Left side of the chest

Heart centre

Navel centre

Lower abdomen

Right hip

Left hip

Right knee

Left knee

Right ankle

Left ankle

Right big toe

Second toe

Third toe

Fourth toe

Little toe

Left big toe

Second toe

Third toe

Fourth toe

Little toe

Be aware of the whole right side of the body

As you sweep awareness through the whole right side of the body, you sweep energy through the whole right side of the body (pause)

Be aware of the whole left side of the body

As you sweep awareness through the whole left side of the body, you sweep energy through the whole left side of the body (pause)

Now be aware of the whole body together

The whole body together

Awareness diffused over the whole body, infusing energy through the whole body.

Diffused awareness, infusing energy.

Effortless. (pause)

Refreshed by the energy of your own awareness. (long pause)

Breath Awareness

Feel as if the whole body is breathing. (long pause)

The whole body, alive with energy.

The whole body, surrounded by energy.

Inhaling and exhaling with the whole body.

No need to change the breath in any way.

Natural breath. Simply observe.

Inhaling and exhaling with the whole body. (long pause)

Feel the exchange of energy – cosmic energy from all around you coming in with each inhale.

Energy within you being shared as you exhale.

Continue to watch this exchange.

Energy in, energy out.

Unlimited energy.

Breathing with the whole body.

Full access to infinite energy all around you.

Every pore of your being drawing it in with each inhale. (pause)

Allow awareness of your body to diffuse even more.

Notice the energy flows in with even more ease as you diffuse awareness. (pause)

Drawing in infinite energy.

Effortless.

The more effortless, the more energy flows through. (pause)

Breathing in this way for just a few more breaths.

Energy in, energy out.

Effortless.

Simply observe. (long pause)

Symbols/Visualization

Continuing to be the witness as you dive into the wellspring of infinite beauty within you.

A treasure trove of creativity, ideas and wisdom.

All your own.

Already within you, accessible anytime.

Familiar symbols will be named. Images or feelings might or might not arise. Both are fine.

Nothing to do but be the witness, like watching a movie screen.

Simply watching, with curiosity and wonder. (pause)

A bright pink daisy (repeat 3 times)

A bowl of bright, yellow lemons (repeat 3 times)

A violet sunset (repeat 3 times)

Sparkling water (repeat 3 times)

Gleaming gold coins (repeat 3 times)

Vast green fields (repeat 3 times)

A fluffy white bunny (repeat 3 times)

Clear blue sky (repeat 3 times)

(pause)

If any insights, ideas, memories or inspiration came to you, you can come back to that later. If not, that's fine too. Know this time has been useful in stimulating your creative capacities whether or not you're aware of it.

Sankalpa

Now, if it feels good, coming back to your sankalpa or the affirmation: "I am vibrant". Allow the feeling to arise in your awareness. (long pause)

Repeat your sankalpa or "I am vibrant" three times, mentally. (long pause)

Take a moment now to feel the joy of your sankalpa already manifesting. (long pause)

If you'd like to continue visualizing your sankalpa manifested, then do.

If you'd like to dive deeper, bring awareness to the point between the eyebrows. Awareness moving to the point between the eyebrows. Not as a physical point of flesh and bone, but as a centre of consciousness.

There is expansion, limitlessness here. Still, silent, limitless. (long pause)

If it feels peaceful, and freeing, allow your awareness to dive into that limitless expanse for the next several minutes. (pause for 2-10 minutes)

Externalization

Ommmmm...

Bring your awareness back to the point between the eyebrows. If the mind has wandered off, that's fine.

Simply bring your awareness back to the point between the eyebrows. (long pause)

Now allow awareness to move down to the nostrils.

Notice the breath moving in and out of the nostrils. (long pause)

Move awareness down further, to the heart centre.

Bring your awareness to your heart centre. (pause)

Notice the heart centre rising on inhalation, falling on exhalation. (pause)

Take a deep breath in, notice awareness coming back to your body.

Awareness rising to the surface, coming back to your body.

Deep breath bringing the energy back to the surface of awareness. Back to awareness of the body.

Feel the movement of the deep breaths breaking up the stillness.

Yoga Nidra is now complete. (pause)

Feel your whole body – legs, arms, back, head, resting on the surface beneath you. (pause)

Notice my voice in the room. (pause)

Notice yourself in the room. (pause)

Wiggle your fingers and toes. Feel them alive with energy.

Bring more energy to the body by stretching or moving however you like. Feel energy alive in the body. (pause)

And if you're lying down, when you're ready, roll to your right side. Take a few deep breaths here. Recalling your practice of bringing vibrancy to the surface, to shine through freely and easily. (long pause)

And if you like, repeating your sankalpa or "I am vibrant", one more time.

If you were lying down, keep your eyes closed if you can and slowly press yourself up to sitting. Take a deep breath. Notice the energy rising as you sit upright. (long pause)

> Option 1: We'll finish by chanting **Om** three times and Shanti three times. Feel the energy rise with the chant. And after a pause in silence, open your eyes when you're ready, allowing your vibrancy shine through, brightly and effortlessly.

(Chant Om Om Om Shanti Shanti Shanti then pause for silence.)

Option 2:

We'll finish by chanting **Om Haum Joom Saha**, an energy-giving mantra. These are not words, they're energies encased in a sound structure. Feel the energy rise with the chant. And after a pause in silence, open your eyes when you're ready, allowing your vibrancy shine through, brightly and effortlessly.

(Chant Om Haum Joom Saha as many times as you like, then pause for silence.)

The Getaway *(30 min.)*

Escape on a glorious getaway. You name the place. Let's go!

Suggested Pre- and Post-Practices:

- This practice assumes participants already have a personal sankalpa. If you have participants new to sankalpa, start with a brief explanation or the Guided Sankalpa Setting from the first Yoga Nidra Scripts book.
- Prepare and/or finish with some basic movements of the joints or simple stretches.
- Begin or finish with a few minutes of holding Anjali Mudra for heart-centred awareness.

Settling

Lying down comfortably, or sitting, supported.

Maybe for today, choosing a position where the heart feels open. Open for this getaway to make your heart sing.

Whatever position you choose, as always, listen to your body to check what feels right.

Cushion your head with a pillow or folded blanket.

Cover yourself with a blanket if you like.

Maybe a soothing scarf over your eyes.

Listening in. What would allow you to feel more free? (pause)

Adjusting just as you'd like. There's no rush. Take your time. (long pause for settling)

And now settling in.

Taking a pause from the busyness of your day.

Headed for a well-deserved getaway.

Travelling first class, in the ultra comfort you've created for yourself.

Going on a getaway, just for you.

Check that everything is just right. (pause)

Are your feet and legs comfortable? (pause)

Hips comfortable? (pause)

What about your back? Is your whole back comfortable? (pause)

Check in with the arms and hands. (pause)

Shoulders. (pause)

Neck. (pause)

Jaw, tongue, forehead. (pause)

The whole body, as comfortable as can be.

Travelling first class. (pause)

And if it feels delightful, melt into that luxurious support. (pause)

Leaving all your cares behind.

Nothing else you need to attend to.

Attention is drawing inward. Into your own sweet self. (pause)

Inhale, taking in the sweetness of this moment.

Exhale letting go into the comfort.

Inhale feeling grateful for this getaway.

Exhale releasing into the comfort, even more. (pause)

Allow your sense of hearing to extend out, receiving sounds, but without analyzing. Simply receiving. Receiving any sounds. (pause)

The farthest sounds (long pause)

Near sounds (long pause)

Maybe even the sound of your own breath. (long pause)

Become aware of the body.

Be aware of your body resting in the luxurious comfort you created. (pause)

Feel stillness in your body.

If at any time you need to move, then move.

Otherwise, you're free to settle in to the comfort.

Free to rest the body.

In luxurious comfort.

Just as you like it.

Just for you.

Effortless. (pause)

Body rests, while awareness is free to travel on. (pause)

Yoga Nidra has now begun. (pause)

Sankalpa

Now if you'd like, allow the joyful feeling of your sankalpa to arise.

Really feel your sankalpa. Picture it vividly. Picture yourself experiencing it. (long pause)

If you took a getaway, to someplace where you could fully experience the joy of your sankalpa manifested, where would that be? (pause)

A place where you can fully revel in the beautiful feeling of your manifested sankalpa.

It could be anywhere. Is it a beach, a cottage, a room in a home, a place of beauty or interest? It can be any place you like, remembered or imagined.

Picture this getaway where you can fully experience your manifested sankalpa. Picture yourself there, as vividly as you can. (long pause)

What do you see? (long pause)

What are the colours? (long pause)

What is the quality of light? (long pause)

What does it sound like? (long pause)

What does it taste like? (long pause)

What does it feel like? (long pause)

Picture it in great detail. See yourself experiencing it. (long pause)

And now, state your sankalpa mentally, three times with confidence and joy. (long pause)

And now, in this beautiful place, begin looking for a quiet, private place to rest, where you can practice your Yoga Nidra body awareness. Look for a place to rest, and go there. (long pause)

Rotation of Consciousness

Now settled in this comfy place, you can begin the process of refreshing the body with energy.

Several energetic points will be named.

Allow awareness to travel freely from point to point.

No need to think or analyze, simply allow awareness to skip from one point to the next.

Where awareness goes, energy flows. Automatically, without effort.

Start with awareness of the right hand.

As awareness moves to the right hand, energy flows to the right hand. Automatically, without doing anything else.

No need to think.

Now move awareness to the left hand

As awareness moves to the left hand, energy effortlessly follows.

Now to the right wrist

Energy follows

The left wrist

Right elbow

Left elbow

Right shoulder

Left shoulder

Hollow of the throat

Back of the head near the top

Crown of the head

Eyebrow centre

Right eyebrow

Left eyebrow

Right eye

Left eye

Right ear

Left ear

Right cheek

Left cheek

Tip of the nose

Upper lip

Lower lip

Tip of the chin

Hollow of the throat

Heart centre

Right side of the chest

Heart centre

Left side of the chest

Heart centre

Navel centre

Lower abdomen

Right hip

Left hip

Right knee

Left knee

Right ankle

Left ankle

Right toes

Left toes

Now the whole right side of the body (pause)

The whole left side of the body (pause)

The whole body together

The whole body together

The whole body together (pause)

The whole body, refreshed with energy. (pause)

Breath Awareness

Now become aware of the breath.

No need to change the breath in any way, simply bring awareness to the breath.

Bring awareness to the natural inhalation.

No changes needed. Just watching.

With each inhale, know that you're drawing in energy.

Drawing in refreshment. Nourishment.

Know that effortlessly, naturally, you're filling up with juicy energy.

Lovely, juicy energy.

Feel that juiciness reaching every cell of your body. (pause)

Refreshing. Nourishing.

All of it happening effortlessly.

With each inhale, naturally drawing in energy.

All of your cells doing a happy dance. Energized with juicy energy.

Refreshed. Nourished. Juicy. (pause)

If it feels good, taking a minute now to continue watching the natural breath in this way, or in any way that feels right. (pause for 1 minute)

Symbols/Visualization

Now getting ready to engage in your getaway again, leaving your resting place.

Getting ready to fully immerse yourself in the experience of your glorious getaway.

Allow your sankalpa to arise. (pause)

Recalling the getaway you experienced earlier. The place where you can fully experience the joy of your manifested sankalpa. (pause)

Visualize yourself back in that place now. (long pause)

This place is your destiny. The place to experience the fulfillment of your sankalpa. (long pause)

Recall all of the details of this place, in living colour. Maybe even discovering new, delightful details. Feel free to explore and immerse.

What do you see? (long pause)

Are there particular sounds? (long pause)

Are there any special foods or drinks you're enjoying? (long pause)

What does it feel like? (long pause)

Picture it in great detail.

See yourself experiencing this incredible getaway.

What are you doing? (long pause)

How are you feeling? (long pause)

Take a minute to enjoy yourself here. (pause for 1 minute)

And now return to your resting place or find a new one.

Return to your resting place or find a new one.

Go to a comfortable space where you can rest, reflect and enjoy a quiet moment to just take it all in. (long pause)

Resting comfortably now, take a moment to recall the events that led up to this experience of your manifested sankalpa, your sankalpa brought to life. What happened along the way to bring you to this joyful destiny? (long pause)

Did you take any actions to get here? (long pause)

Did you shift your mindset at all, to arrive here? (long pause)

Was there anything you needed to gain or anything you needed to release to be here, sankalpa manifested? (long pause)

Were there others you connected with for help? (long pause)

Reflecting on anything that might have happened for you to be able to be here now, at this glorious getaway, experiencing the joy of your manifested sankalpa. (long pause)

Taking a moment of gratitude for yourself or anyone else who might have helped you to get here. (long pause)

And now, moving from this restful space back into the heart of your getaway. Looking out at this beautiful experience. Taking it all in. (long pause)

Feeling the experience, take a moment to state your sankalpa mentally, three times with full confidence and joy. (long pause)

And now, feeling refreshed and inspired after this glorious getaway, know that it's time to return your awareness back to your body. Excited to return to the body and enjoy the journey toward your manifested sankalpa. That journey has already begun. And you can return to your glorious getaway to renew your inspiration, anytime you need. (pause)

Externalization

Bringing awareness slowly back to the body, become aware of your breath. (pause)

Your body resting, breathing itself. (pause)

Hear the sound of your body breathing. (long pause)

Feel the sensation of your body breathing. (pause)

Shifting from internal awareness to external awareness.

Yoga Nidra practice is coming to an end.

Take a deep breath and feel awareness coming back into the body. (pause)

Yoga Nidra is now complete. (pause)

Begin to gently move the body. Wiggle fingers and toes. Roll your ankles and wrists around. Waking back up, into the body.

Stretch your body in ways that feel refreshing, then when you're ready, if you were lying down, roll to the right side. (long pause)

Take a few deep breaths, recalling your experience at your getaway. The experience of your sankalpa brought to life. (long pause)

If you like, repeat your sankalpa one more time, fully aware of the power it holds to change your life in amazing ways. (long pause)

And now, if you were lying down, with eyes closed if possible, gently, mindfully press yourself up to sitting, without disturbing the body too much. (long pause)

Sitting comfortably, back as straight as you can make it.

Take a deep breath in… and a long breath out.

Hold any positive feelings you had at your getaway. (long pause)

We'll finish by chanting Om and Shanti, three times each.

Take a deep breath in.

Om Om Om Shanti Shanti Shanti (pause)

Refreshed and excited to be on this journey as your sankalpa develops into beautiful new realities, open your eyes.

In The Loving Arms of Mother Earth
(30-35 min.)

Surrender any worry, nervousness or feelings of ungroundedness, into the loving arms of Mother Earth.

Suggested Pre- and Post-Practices:

- Begin with gentle movements that release tension from the joints and/or major muscles. Consider adding grounding movements like squatting, seated poses, child's pose – keeping the arms down and shoulders relaxed. Also consider movements that release tension from the shoulders, neck and lower back.

- Prepare or finish with a few minutes of Hridaya Mudra, Abhaya Hridaya Mudra, or Anjali Mudra to connect with the spiritual heart.

- Prepare or finish with any Goddess Mantra, or prayer to the Divine Mother.

Settling

Getting ready to leave any worry, nervous energy, ungroundedness behind.

Lying in savasana or sitting supported.

If you're lying down and have any tension in the low back, place a pillow or bolster under your knees, maybe something soft under your heels.

Choosing a soft, folded blanket or cushion to support your neck and head. Maybe tucking it in around the sides of your head to give you a cradled sensation if that feels good.

Listening in to your body to hear what it's asking for, then without hesitation, giving your body exactly what it needs in this moment.

Doing whatever you need to do to be as comfortable as possible.

If it's difficult to relax, that's fine too. You're welcome just as you are. Simply create as much comfort as you can, as best as you can. (long pause for settling)

And now, scanning the body. Be aware of any areas that feel tense. (pause)

Is there an adjustment you could make to feel more comfortable? Make any adjustments that are helpful. (long pause)

Making any final adjustments now. Settling into the comfort. (pause)

Take a deep breath in, and as you exhale, surrender to gravity. (pause)

Take another deep breath in, and exhale, release into the comfort.

Settling into these moments for rest.

Moments to feel supported and cared for.

Moments to connect with the loving energy of Mother Earth. (pause)

In this comfort, begin to notice the sensation of effortlessness arising. (pause)

Body becoming effortless.

Senses turning inward, resting.

You might even feel as if you can receive these words with effortless awareness. (pause)

Comfortable.

Resting.

Effortless.

Yoga Nidra has now begun. (pause)

Sankalpa

And now, if you already have a sankalpa, allow the joyful feeling of it to arise. If you don't have a sankalpa, you can use "I am calm". (pause)

Really feel your sankalpa, picture it – as vividly as you can. (long pause)

If the feeling is there, it can't help but be manifested.

State your sankalpa, or "I am calm", mentally with feeling, three times now. (long pause)

Rotation of Consciousness

Now moving awareness through the body from point to point.

Nothing you need to accomplish or experience.

No way to get this wrong.

Awareness is effortless.

Start by becoming aware of the right side of the body

Not looking for anything, simply be aware of the right side of the body

Now become aware of the right hand

Right hand thumb

Index finger

Middle finger

Ring finger

Little finger

Awareness moving effortlessly

Palm of the hand

Back of the hand

Right wrist

Lower arm

Elbow

Upper arm

Shoulder

Armpit

Right side of the ribs

Right side of the waist

Right hip

Right thigh

Knee

Lower leg

Ankle

Heel

Sole of the foot

Top of the foot

Right big toe

Second toe

Third toe

Fourth toe

Fifth toe

Awake and aware

Move awareness to the left side of the body

Become aware of the left hand

Left hand thumb

Index finger

Middle finger

Ring finger

Little finger

Palm of the hand

Back of the hand

Left wrist

Lower arm

Elbow

Upper arm

Shoulder

Armpit

Left side of the ribs

Left side of the waist

Left hip

Left thigh

Knee

Lower leg

Ankle

Heel

Sole of the foot

Top of the foot

Left big toe

Second toe

Third toe

Fourth toe

Fifth toe

Awake and aware

Move awareness up to the crown of the head

Crown of the head

Forehead

Right temple

Left temple

Right eyebrow

Left eyebrow

Eyebrow centre

Right eye

Left eye

Right ear

Left ear

Right cheek

Left cheek

Right nostril

Left nostril

Upper lip

Lower lip

Chin

Throat centre

Right collarbone

Left collarbone

Right side of the chest

Left side of the chest

Heart centre

Navel

Lower abdomen

Move awareness to the back of the body

Sacrum

Lower back

Middle back

Upper back

Right shoulder blade

Left shoulder blade

Back of the neck

Back of the head

Crown of the head

Move awareness all the way down to the whole right leg

The whole left leg

Both legs together

The whole torso

The whole right arm

The whole left arm

Both arms together

Neck

Head

The whole front of the body

The whole back of the body

Become aware of the whole body together

The whole body together

The whole body together (long pause)

Breath Awareness

Become aware of your natural breath. (pause)

Soft. Effortless. (pause)

Be aware of the exhalation. (long pause)

As you exhale, feel as if any worries, nervousness, ungroundedness is moving down and out. (pause)

Follow the exhalation, down and out. (pause)

Feel that with each exhalation, more of the worry, nervousness, ungroundedness is moving down and out. (pause)

Exhale, worry, nervousness, ungroundedness, down and out.

Feel that with each exhale you begin to feel more grounded, more settled, more calm. (pause)

Each exhale, more grounded, settled, calm. (pause)

Exhaling down and out, becoming grounded, settled, calm. (pause)

Keep following this breath for the next minute. (pause for 1 minute)

Symbols/Visualization

Following this feeling of groundedness, if it feels good, allow an image of a beautiful, completely private plot of earth to arise in your awareness. A beautiful place where you'd like to lie down, right on the earth, to take a load off and simply rest.

It might be a warm, private sandy beach, a grassy field, a drift of powdery snow – any place that feels soothing and sublimely comfortable. (pause)

It could be a place you've visited or an imaginary place. There's no limitation. It's completely up to you. A place all to yourself where you can just sink in, right on the earth and feel at ease. (pause)

A beautiful, natural spot where you feel completely welcome. Allow this comforting place to arise in your awareness now.(long pause)

And now, nestle into this beautiful, natural plot of earth. (long pause)

Here you are, at home.

In the loving arms of Mother Earth.

Nothing asked of you.

You can simply be.

Welcome in all ways.

Just as you are.

You are a child of Mother Earth.

Welcome in every way, and at every moment. Lying here, know that Mother Earth is always here to comfort you. (long pause)

Always here to comfort you. (pause)

Gaze at her dazzling night sky and know she's always here to inspire you. (long pause)

Always here to inspire you. (pause)

Rest in the light of her setting sun to know she is always here to soothe and calm you. (long pause)

Always here to soothe and calm you. (pause)

You are a child of Mother Earth.

You are welcome in every way, every aspect of your being, at every moment. You are cared for and supported at every moment.

You can surrender your worries, your challenges and know her mighty strength will carry you.

You are in the loving arms of Mother Earth.

At every moment.

In the loving arms of Mother Earth, taking a minute now to rest. Simply rest. (pause for 1 minute)

Sankalpa

While you're nestled here, in the loving arms of Mother Earth, allow your sankalpa, or "I am calm" to arise in your awareness.

In the loving arms of Mother Earth, whisper to her this heart's desire, this sankalpa. (long pause)

She's excited to hear your heart's desire, and can't wait to help you make your beautiful sankalpa a beautiful reality. Know that she is always conspiring to help you move in the direction of your dreams. (pause)

Feel that love and care from Mother Earth.

Love, care, support.

Rest now in that love, care and support, in the loving arms of Mother Earth, for the next few minutes. (pause for 2-5 minutes)

Externalization

Ommmmmmmm

Bring awareness back to your beautiful, natural plot of earth, feeling thankful for your experience. (pause)

Getting ready to say goodbye, knowing you can return to this experience in the loving arms of Mother Earth anytime. (pause)

In any way you like, take a moment to say goodbye and prepare to leave. (long pause)

And now bring awareness back into your body.

Feel your body comfortably resting.

Notice your body resting in the comfort you created. (pause)

Take a deep breath in, and a long breath out, bringing awareness back to your body. (pause)

Awareness coming back to the body now.

Yoga Nidra is now complete. (pause)

Begin to move the body by wiggling your fingers and toes.

Stretch or move in any way that feels good. Any way that makes you feel energized back in the body and yet calmer than when you began. (long pause)

And if you're lying down, when you're ready, roll to your right side.

Take a few deep breaths and recall your experience in the loving arms of Mother Earth. The support. The care. The love. Or any positive experience you had. (long pause)

And if you like, repeat your sankalpa or "I am calm", mentally one more time, feeling its increased strength, now nourished by Mother Earth. (long pause)

If you were lying down, press yourself up to sitting, eyes closed, feeling grounded and with renewed strength. (long pause)

Take a deep breath. (pause)

We'll finish by chanting Om three times and Shanti three times. You can join in if you like or simply enjoy the soothing vibration. If you're joining in, take a deep breath in. (pause)

Om Om Om Shanti Shanti Shanti (pause)

Bringing any positive sensations from your practice into the rest of your day. When you're ready, open your eyes.

Sacred Pilgrimage *(30-40 min.)*

Take a pilgrimage to a sacred site to deliver an offering and receive spiritual guidance.

Suggested Pre- and Post-Practices:
- This practice assumes participants already have a personal sankalpa. If you have participants new to sankalpa, start with a brief explanation or the Guided Sankalpa Setting from the first Yoga Nidra Scripts book.
- Prepare with a few minutes of Yoni Mudra for receptivity and improving intuition. Or a meditative mudra such as Bhairava or Bhairavi Mudra.
- Prepare and/or finish with some basic movements of the joints or simple stretches.
- Begin with a prayer or liberation mantra, for example:

  Asato Ma Sat Gamaya

  Tamaso Ma Jyotir Gamaya

  Mrityor Ma Amritam Gamaya

  Om Shanti Shanti Shanti

  (Lead me from the unreal to the real, darkness to light, death to immortality)

Settling

Getting ready to lie down comfortably or sit up, supported. Gathering any props you need.

Getting set up so you can fall into a deep relaxation.

Taking a folded blanket or cushion under your head, maybe something under your knees to add comfort to your lower back, a blanket to cover you, a scarf over your eyes… anything you need that will make your body sigh, ahhhhh. (long pause)

Getting ready for this Yoga Nidra practice that will take you on a spiritual pilgrimage.

In the spirit of this sacred journey, treat your body with reverence as you are setting yourself up. Treat your body as a temple.

Listening in now with care and reverence, offering your body anything it needs in this moment.

Listening carefully, and acting as a loving servant to your body. (long pause for settling)

Now ask your body if it's completely comfortable. (pause)

Make any adjustments needed. (long pause)

Feel your body begin to release into the comfort.

Body fully supported, effortlessly dropping into a state of peace.

Body effortlessly dropping into a state of non-doing.

Letting go of doing.

Shifting, into being.

Notice the sensation of your body releasing tension in the shoulders. (pause)

Releasing tensions in the back. (pause)

The arms. (pause)

The legs. (pause)

Completely releasing tension.

Body is still and at ease.

See your body, as if from above – resting, breathing, peacefully. (pause)

The body rests, while the awareness continues on.

Become aware of the soft sound of the body breathing itself. (long pause)

Effortless breathing, effortless awareness.

Awake.

Aware.

Effortless.

Yoga Nidra has now begun. (pause)

Sankalpa

Allow your sankalpa to arise in your awareness. (pause)

Allow the feeling of your sankalpa to arise. (pause)

Vividly see your sankalpa manifested. (long pause)

Feel your sankalpa manifested. (long pause)

And now, repeat your sankalpa with joy, three times mentally. (long pause)

Know with certainty, that your sankalpa is now stored within you like a blueprint. Your whole being is now following its direction, conspiring to create beautiful new realities at every moment. (pause)

Rotation of Consciousness

Now moving awareness through the body from point to point.

Experiencing energetically, awareness moving freely, without attachment.

Begin with effortless awareness of the point between the eyebrows

Effortless awareness of the point between the eyebrows

Moving freely to the hollow of the throat

The right shoulder joint

Elbow joint

Wrist joint

The right thumb

Tip of the index finger

Tip of the middle finger

Tip of the ring finger

Tip of the little finger

Experiencing energetically

The wrist joint

Elbow joint

Shoulder joint

Hollow of the throat

Over to the left shoulder joint

Elbow joint

Wrist joint

The left thumb

Tip of the index finger

Tip of the middle finger

Tip of the ring finger

Tip of the little finger

Back up to the wrist joint

Elbow joint

Shoulder joint

Hollow of the throat

The heart centre

The right side of the chest

The heart centre

The left side of the chest

The heart centre

The navel centre

The lower abdomen

The right hip joint

Right knee joint

Ankle joint

The right big toe

Tip of the second toe

Tip of the third toe

Tip of the fourth toe

Tip of the baby toe

Back up to the right ankle joint

Knee joint

Hip joint

Sweeping awareness to the left hip joint

Left knee joint

Ankle joint

The left big toe

Tip of the second toe

Tip of the third toe

Tip of the fourth toe

Tip of the baby toe

Back up to the left ankle joint

Knee joint

Hip joint

The lower abdomen

The navel centre

The heart centre

Hollow of the throat

The eyebrow centre

The eyebrow centre

The eyebrow centre (pause)

Breath Awareness

Feel as if you are breathing in and out of the point between the eyebrows.

Effortlessly breathing in and out of the point between the eyebrows. (long pause)

Breathing in and out of the point between the eyebrows.

This is the gateway of knowledge and intuition. (long pause)

Be aware of any subtle sensations. (pause)

Breathing in and out of the point between the eyebrows. (long pause)

Symbols/Visualization

Now if it feels right, allowing awareness to travel on, embarking on a sacred pilgrimage.

Taking a pilgrimage to a place that stirs your spiritual heart.

A place where you feel connected to a higher power.

A place of awe and beauty. That stirs your spiritual heart. (pause)

Allow such a place to arise in your awareness now. It might be a place you've been, a place you've dreamed of going to, or an imagined place. A holy site, a place of natural beauty, any place that has spiritual significance to you. Allow it to arise in your awareness now. (long pause)

Prepare to travel to this special place, but before you go, if it feels right, choose an offering to bring with you. Something special you'd like to take on your spiritual pilgrimage, to give as an offering when you're there. It might be an item, a promise, a prayer.

If you'd like, take a moment now to choose a heart-felt offering, to take with you on your sacred pilgrimage. (long pause)

And now embarking on the journey, with joyful anticipation.

See yourself travelling to your sacred site now. You can travel in any way you like. (pause)

Notice the sights along the way... the sounds... the scents. Vividly experience your journey to your sacred site. (long pause)

If you haven't yet arrived at your place of pilgrimage, now is the time to arrive. (pause)

As you arrive, you are in awe. It is a place of such beauty and your joy can hardly be contained. (pause)

Allow all of your senses to take in this sacred place. To be fully present in the experience.

Notice the light, the colours. (long pause)

Notice the sounds. (long pause)

Notice any scents. (long pause)

Notice any sensations. (long pause)

With great humility, you approach an area of special significance to you.

It's as if it's calling your name. It's as if it's been waiting for this opportunity to connect with you. (long pause)

You approach closely and know this is the moment for your offering.

If you have an offering, take a moment now, with great reverence, to give your offering. (long pause)

Feel the joy of giving the offering, and the joy in knowing it's been received. (long pause)

Take a moment in gratitude for this precious opportunity to connect with the Divine. (long pause)

If you'd like to ask for any spiritual guidance, speak from your heart, say a prayer, or simply enjoy the peace and comfort here, in this sacred place, take time to do that now. (pause for 1 minute)

If it feels right, give gratitude once more, from deep in your heart, for the opportunity to be heard, receive guidance or simply be here, feeling the presence of the Divine. (long pause)

Sankalpa

Finally, before you go, share your beloved sankalpa. From deep in your heart. Repeat your sankalpa in the presence of this holy energy, in this sacred place, three times now, with full feeling and awareness. (long pause)

Feel that the sankalpa has been blessed by Divine grace. (pause)

Feel the gratitude swell, deep in your heart. (pause)

Before leaving this sacred place, find a place to sit in quiet reflection. To sit for meditation. (long pause)

Sitting for meditation, allow your awareness to travel deep into the heart centre. Deep into the sacred cave of your heart. (pause)

Traveling deep, past the emotional heart, deep into the peace of the spiritual heart.

Tranquil. Calm. Comforting. (pause)

The cave of your heart.

The sacred cave of your heart. (pause)

Effortless. Peaceful.

Resting here, in the sacred cave of your heart, with full awareness for the next several minutes. (pause 4-10 minutes)

Externalization

Ommmmmmmm

Bring awareness back to the heart centre if your mind has wandered off. (pause)

Coming back out of your meditation, it's time to leave this sacred place of pilgrimage.

Say goodbye, taking the positive memories of your experience with you. You can return again any time you like. (long pause)

See yourself travelling away from your sacred site now. You can travel in any way you like. Notice the sights along the way... the sounds… the scents. Vividly experience your journey returning back to your resting body. (long pause)

If your awareness hasn't yet arrived back in your body, back in the room, now is the time. (pause)

Awareness returning back to the room.

Awareness coming back into your body.

Beginning to notice sensations in the physical body.

Notice the chest rising and falling with each breath.

Feel the chest rising and falling with each breath. (pause)

Yoga Nidra is now complete. (pause)

Taking a few deep breaths now and notice sensation coming back to the body. (long pause)

Wiggle your fingers and toes.

Stretch your body out.

Feel awareness coming back into the body. (long pause)

If you're lying down, when you're ready, roll to your right side.

Take a few deep breaths. (long pause)

If you like, mentally repeat your sankalpa one more time. Feel it fill your whole being. (long pause)

Remember your sacred pilgrimage and any guidance, experiences or reflections you had that you'd like to carry forward. (long pause)

Keep your eyes closed if you can, and if you were lying down, press yourself up to sitting.

Take as much time as you need. (long pause)

Take a few deep breaths in. (long pause)

We'll finish by chanting Om and Shanti three times each.

Take a deep breath in.

Om Om Om Shanti Shanti Shanti (pause)

Carrying any positive feelings from your heart-felt pilgrimage with you.

When you're ready, open your eyes.

Expanding Identity *(35-40 min.)*

Feeling stuck? You might be holding onto an identity that's limiting you. Reconnect with the truth that you are free.

Suggested Pre- and Post-Practices:

- Prepare of finish with stretches that move the spine in all ways – forward, back, side and twisting.
- Prepare with a few minutes of chanting Om, while holding Chin Mudra or any meditative mudra to connect with the nature of the Self.
- Prepare with Breath of Joy pranayama to lift the spirit and energy.
- Begin with a mantra that speaks to the nature of the Self, such as:

    Asato Ma Sat Gamaya

    Tamaso Ma Jyotir Gamaya

    Mrityor Ma Amritam Gamaya

    Om Shanti Shanti Shanti (pause)

    (Lead me from the unreal to the real, darkness to light, death to immortality)

Settling

Preparing for your Yoga Nidra practice. Lying on your back, side, or sitting up, supported.

Getting ready for this practice for reconnecting with your essential freedom.

Maybe making a cozy rest nest with cushions, blankets, bolsters – whatever your body needs to feel as comfortable as possible in this moment. (long pause for settling)

Getting comfortable for this practice of non-doing.

If there are any adjustments you need so you can more easily sink into the comfort, make them now. (pause)

Getting ready to do nothing. (pause)

Nothing you need to do.

Nothing you need to be.

Nothing you need to feel.

No one you need to please.

There is only you.

Experiencing this practice in any way you like.

From any perspective you like.

Reconnecting with your essential freedom. (pause)

There's no way to get this wrong.

Simply enjoy the ride. (pause)

Check in with how you feel.

Check that your feet and ankles are comfortable. (pause)

Calves, knees and thighs comfortable. (pause)

Hips comfortable. (pause)

Lower back, middle back, upper back comfortable. Whole back, melting. (pause)

Hands and arms relax. (pause)

Shoulders and neck relax. (pause)

Jaw, tongue and cheeks soften. (pause)

Eyes, forehead and scalp soften. (pause)

Whole body, completely released into the comfort. (pause)

You can move anytime you like, but if it feels good, enjoy the stillness. (long pause)

Be aware of the room you're in. The size of the room, ceiling, walls... any artwork... any furniture... the colour of the floor... the space around you... (pause)

Feel the temperature of the props your using. (pause) Feel the temperature on your face. (pause)

Be aware of sounds, far away. Not identifying the sounds. Simply be aware of the sounds. (long pause)

Now be aware of sounds in the room. Not identifying, just receiving. (long pause)

Awareness becoming more and more subtle.

Effortless awareness. (pause)

Simply receiving, without analysis or judgement. (pause)

Simply experiencing, effortlessly. Without naming the things experienced or the experience itself. (pause)

Not naming the things experienced or the experience itself.

Simply experiencing.

Pure experience. (pause)

Yoga Nidra has now begun. (pause)

Sankalpa

Bring awareness to the body.

What is the body? Your whole body is made of food. The food you've eaten has become your muscles, your skin, your brain. Your whole body is made of food. (pause)

That food, is made of carbon. (pause)

That carbon, is stardust. (pause)

Stardust recycled as different forms over and over and over.

So what are you? (pause)

Right now, are you either lying down or sitting? (pause)

Maybe you said, "Yes, I'm lying down, or I'm sitting". When in fact, it is the body that is lying down or sitting. This mass of food, carbon, stardust. (pause)

If you are experiencing the body, you are not the body. You are the one experiencing the body. You are the witness, the awareness. (pause)

If the body is a false label for your identity, are there other false labels you might be holding onto? (pause)

You are the limitless awareness. (pause)

Your essential nature is that you are free. Limitless. Your Soul is limitless. (pause)

Each label or identity on top of this limitless Soul is a limitation.

Are there labels you've accepted or created that are limiting you? Holding you back? (pause)

What labels would you like to expand beyond? (pause)

Is there a career identification, for example, "I am a lawyer"?

Is there a social label "I am an introvert"?

Is there an emotional label, "I am sad"?

Remember, you are essentially free. What labels might you be subscribing to that are keeping you stuck? Keeping you limited? (long pause)

How would you like to expand? You might use this phrase, "Up until now, I was…" Use your own words for the label you'd like to expand beyond. For example, "Up until now, I was an introvert." Use your own words now: "Up until now, I was…" (long pause)

And now choosing a sankalpa that inspires freedom, a message to your Soul to always stay connected to your essential freedom. Maybe, "I am free", or "I am unlimited". Or any other short, memorable, heart-felt statement in your own words. Choosing your sankalpa now. (long pause)

Allow the positive feeling, and expansive quality of your chosen sankalpa to grow. Feel the unlimited potential. (long pause)

And now, repeat your chosen sankalpa or "I am free", or "I am unlimited", mentally, three times. (long pause)

Know that this expansive sankalpa has made a lasting impression and has already begun to create positive change in your life.

Rotation of Consciousness

Now bring your awareness back to the body.

Though it is stardust, it is *your* beautiful stardust. Your body is your vehicle for experiencing this life, and deserves your tender loving care and attention.

Moving awareness through the body now.

Effortless awareness, moving from point to point.

Sensations, experiences, thoughts might arise as awareness moves, simply notice and move on.

Start by bringing awareness to the point between the eyebrows

Effortless awareness of the point between the eyebrows

The hollow of the throat

The right shoulder joint

Elbow joint

Wrist joint

The right thumb

The tip of the index finger

Tip of the middle finger

Tip of the ring finger

Tip of the little finger

The right wrist joint

Elbow joint

Shoulder joint

Hollow of the throat

Over to the left shoulder joint

Elbow joint

Wrist joint

The left thumb

Tip of the index finger

Tip of the middle finger

Tip of the ring finger

Tip of the little finger

Back up to the left wrist joint

Elbow joint

Shoulder joint

Hollow of the throat

The heart centre

The right side of the chest

The heart centre

The left side of the chest

The heart centre

The navel centre

Lower abdomen

The right hip joint

Right knee joint

Ankle joint

The right big toe

Tip of the second toe

Tip of the third toe

Tip of the fourth toe

Tip of the baby toe

Back up to the right ankle joint

Knee joint

Hip joint

Sweeping awareness to the left hip joint

Left knee joint

Ankle joint

The left big toe

Tip of the second toe

Tip of the third toe

Tip of the fourth toe

Tip of the baby toe

Back up to the left ankle joint

Knee joint

Hip joint

Lower abdomen

Navel centre

Heart centre

Hollow of the throat

The eyebrow centre

The eyebrow centre

The eyebrow centre (pause)

Breath Awareness

Feel as if you are breathing in and out through the point between the eyebrows. (pause)

In a straight line, from the point between the eyebrows to the centre of the brain. (long pause)

Breathing like this for several breaths now. (pause for 4-5 breaths)

Allow the breath to become subtle. (pause)

Breathing in a straight line, from the point between the eyebrows to the centre of the brain. (pause)

Breath becoming subtler and subtler. (pause)

Until the breath is almost imperceptible. (long pause)

Sankalpa

Now allowing the sankalpa you chose earlier to arise again.

It might have been "I am free", "I am unlimited", or any other heart-felt statement you chose. (long pause)

Allow the positive feeling, and expansive quality of your chosen sankalpa to grow. Feel the unlimited potential. (long pause)

And now, repeat your sankalpa or "I am free", or "I am unlimited", mentally, three times. (long pause)

Know that this expansive sankalpa has made a lasting impression and has already begun to create positive change in your life. (long pause)

Shifting awareness to the heart centre, resting awareness at the heart centre.

Move awareness deep. Beyond flesh and bone. More subtle. Sensing the spiritual heart.

The unlimited spiritual heart. The heart of your being. Feel the expansive quality here. An expanse of potential.

Diving deep into this expanse of unlimited potential that is the heart, the core, the source of your being.

Unlimited potential. The source of your being.

Freedom.

Peace.

The source of your being.

Resting now in the peace and silence here, for the next several minutes. (pause 5-10 min)

Externalization

Ommmmmm

Bring awareness back to the breath.

Awareness of the breath streaming in and out of the nostrils. (pause)

Be aware of the sound of the breath. (long pause)

Be aware of sounds in the room and beyond. (long pause)

Visualize the room. Visualize your body resting in the room. (long pause)

Awareness coming back to the body.

Take a deep breath in.

Bringing awareness back to the body.

Feel energy and awareness coming back into the body.

Yoga Nidra is now complete. (pause)

Take another deep breath in and a long breath out, becoming more aware of the body. (pause)

Taking a moment of gratitude for the opportunity to have a body. This beautiful stardust, your vehicle for experiencing this life. (pause)

Give it the tender loving care it deserves as you wake back up into the body, stretching and moving in any way that feels good. (long pause)

And if you're lying down, roll to the right side.

If you like, take a moment to recall any positive or interesting experiences from your Yoga Nidra practice today. Or if you fell asleep, that's fine too. Your body needed the sleep. Either way, it's win-win. Recalling any positive experience or insight, or simply enjoy the sensation of rest. (long pause)

Mindfully make your way to sitting upright.

Keeping eyes closed if you can.

Feel energy rising as you sit.

Feel the body activating.

Mind activating.

And yet, still remaining relaxed. (long pause)

And before we finish, take another moment to repeat your sankalpa if you like, feeling inspired by the realization that you are essentially free, and unlimited. (long pause)

I'll finish by chanting Om and Shanti three times each. Join in if you like.

Notice the energy rise with the chant.

Take a deep breath in.

Om Om Om Shanti Shanti Shanti (pause)

Reconnected with your essential freedom, when you're ready, softly reopen your eyes.

Summer Meadow *(35-45 min.)*

Enjoy a beautiful experience of interconnectedness, nourishment and personal growth – from a whole new perspective.

Suggested Pre- and Post-Practices:

- Begin with a few minutes of Yoni Mudra for receiving prana.
- Finish with a prana-giving mantra, such as:
  Om Haum Joom Saha.

Settling

Getting ready for your Yoga Nidra practice.

This is time for you to rest, connect, discover.

Right now, take some time to build a comfortable rest nest for yourself, whatever that might look like.

Lying on your back in savasana, lying on your side, sitting up, supported… Whatever is best for today, suit yourself, because there's no one else this practice is for. (pause)

You might choose to have a pillow under your head, a blanket covering you, a light eye covering, a bolster or pillow under your knees to ease tension from your lower back…

Choose anything and everything that will help you feel fully supported and as comfortable as possible.

Take the time now to build your ultimate rest nest, with every creature comfort provided. (long pause for settling)

And now that you're settling in, check in.

Do you feel comfortable enough to soften into the support you've built for yourself?

If not, take the time to adjust. If yes, then allow the body to soften, even more. (long pause)

Check that your legs are softening... back softening... arms softening... shoulders... neck... face... the whole body, softening into the comfort you've built for yourself. (pause)

There's no way to do this incorrectly. If you need to make any further adjustments, go ahead and make them. Give yourself full permission to do whatever you need, when you need, so you can settle in comfortably for the beautiful journey of discovery that awaits. (long pause)

And now, once you've done all you can to create this beautiful rest nest for yourself, feel your body softening even more into that support.

Body supported, effortlessly dropping into a state of peace.

Effortlessly dropping into a state of non-doing. (pause)

Nothing to do now.

Letting go of doing.

Shifting into being. (pause)

Feel your body sigh with relief at this opportunity to do nothing. (pause)

This opportunity to rest and renew.

Body is resting, while awareness continues on, free to move and explore.

Allow awareness to explore the space around you. Sensing the size of the space... the light in the space... the objects nearby... the colours... the surface beneath you.

Feel the surface beneath you. (pause)

Exploring awareness of the textures of fabric on your skin. (long pause)

Awareness of the sounds. (long pause)

Awareness of the sound of your own breath. (long pause)

Awake.

Aware.

Effortless awareness. (pause)

Yoga Nidra has now begun. (pause)

Rotation of Consciousness

Moving awareness into the body.

Freely shifting awareness from point to point.

Begin with awareness of the right hand

Nothing you need to think about or do, simply be aware of the right hand

Be aware of the right hand thumb

Right index finger

Middle finger

Ring finger

Little finger

Palm of the hand

Back of the hand

Wrist

Effortless awareness, moving freely up to the right lower arm

Elbow

Upper arm

Shoulder

Armpit

Right side of the ribs

Right side of the waist

Right hip

Right thigh

Right knee

Lower leg

Ankle

Heel

Sole of the foot

Top of the foot

Right big toe

Second toe

Third toe

Fourth toe

Fifth toe

Awake and aware

Sweeping awareness over to the left side of the body now

Be aware of the left hand

Left hand thumb

Index finger

Middle finger

Ring finger

Little finger

Palm of the hand

Back of the hand

Wrist

Moving freely

Left lower arm

Elbow

Upper arm

Shoulder

Armpit

Left side of the ribs

Left side of the waist

Left hip

Left thigh

Left knee

Lower leg

Ankle

Heel

Sole of the foot

Top of the foot

Left big toe

Second toe

Third toe

Fourth toe

Fifth toe

Sweeping awareness up to the crown of the head

Crown of the head

Forehead

Right temple

Left temple

Right eyebrow

Left eyebrow

Eyebrow centre

Right eye

Left eye

Right ear

Left ear

Right cheek

Left cheek

Right nostril

Left nostril

Upper lip

Lower lip

Chin

Throat centre

Right collarbone

Left collarbone

Right side of the chest

Left side of the chest

Heart centre

Navel

Lower abdomen

Sweeping awareness to the back of the body

Sacrum

Lower back

Middle back

Upper back

Right shoulder blade

Left shoulder blade

Back of the neck

Back of the head

Crown of the head

Sweep awareness down to the whole right leg

The whole left leg

Both legs together

The whole torso

The whole right arm

The whole left arm

Both arms and torso, all together

Neck

Head

The whole front of the body (pause)

The whole back of the body (pause)

Become aware of the whole body together

The whole body together

The whole body together (long pause)

Maybe noticing here, that as awareness diffuses to the whole body, your sense of self expands. (pause)

Breath Awareness

Notice this expanded self, breathing.

The whole self, breathing.

Breathing itself.

Nothing to do. (pause)

Take notice for a moment.

With every inhale, your being is effortlessly pulling in energy. (pause)

Your being knows just what to do. (long pause)

Notice the effortless, momentary pause between the inhale and exhale. (long pause)

Something magical happens here – in the pause between the inhale and exhale.

In that split second, your being transforms the incoming energy.

And as you exhale, your unique energetic gift is shared universally. (pause)

Receiving energy and giving energy.

A perfect process.

And your being does this perfectly. And effortlessly.

This is the natural, effortless truth of your being.

As you inhale, you're nourished.

In the pause, transformation.

With the exhale, you nourish.

Inhale, nourished.

Exhale, nourish.

Inhale, nourished.

Exhale, nourish.

Effortlessly, with each breath, your being is receiving and giving.

Automatically.

A beautiful exchange of universal life force. (pause)

Taking a minute now to breathe. You can simply observe the natural breath, or if it feels good, continue to mentally repeat, "Inhale, nourished. Exhale nourish." (pause for 1 minute)

Symbols/Visualization

Now freeing awareness from the breath, to embark on a beautiful journey.

Another perfect process of nourishment and nourishing.

While your body is safely and comfortably resting, your awareness is free to explore. (pause)

You can bring your awareness back to the body anytime you like.

You can also allow your awareness to explore if you like.

Your awareness is free to travel anywhere you like, in any way you like.

So if you'd like, allow your awareness to consider travelling to a lush summer meadow.

Green, floral, warm and inviting.

A vast and private meadow that you share only with the singing birds, hopping bunnies and other friendly flora and fauna. (long pause)

Allow your awareness to seek out an especially lush and inviting area of this vast meadow. (long pause)

Get closer in to see the soft green grasses, and delicate flowers in a multitude of shapes and colours. (long pause)

You're so close, you might even notice some of the fragrance. (pause)

Getting closer still, awareness travels to the roots of the grasses and flowers.

To the rich brown soil. Moist and rich, perfect for growth. You might notice a soothing, earthy scent. (pause)

If you like, allow your awareness to explore even deeper – an inch beneath the soil.

There is a seed there. If it feels good, allow awareness to travel into the seed. (pause)

It's comfy here in this cozy little shell, nestled in the warm earth. Moist and permeable. Soaking up nourishment. (pause)

You feel urged to expand into that inviting warm earth, explore further, take in more nourishment. So you send down a root.

Ah, the deliciousness of stretching out.

And still comfy and cozy in your warm earth bed, in your cozy seed body.

So delightful. (pause)

And then, an idea – you send up a shoot, moving up through the soil, exploring upward, within the soil.

And at the same time, stretching out more roots down in the soil, feasting on nourishment. (pause)

Stretching out, above and below, cozy, warm, nourished and exploring in the soil. (pause)

And then, a beautiful thing…

Light.

Warm sunlight. Toasty. Warmer than the soil.

Your new sprout soaking it in.

And the realization… you are no longer a seed.

Yet you are still you. (pause)

Enjoying new sensations.

The warmth, the breeze, the space. (long pause)

You feel the urge to look up.

You unfurl. Your sprout body opening up, to the sun.

Bright, joyful, ecstatic.

A new type of nourishment.

You dance in your sprout body. Dancing in the sunlight. All day long. (pause)

Following the sun until it slips away.

And then something new – the moon.

Sublime, restful light. And comforting darkness, like the earth you came from.

Coolness, like the earth cradling your now deep roots.

Day after day, this cycle repeats.

Sunrise, daylight, sunset, moonlight.

And each cycle your roots grow deeper, you expand more leaves, you grow taller, closer to the sun, you take more nourishment, from above and below.

Reveling in nourishment. (pause)

Then one day, a tiny bud.

Something new, but familiar. Cozy, like when you were a seed.

Bud getting larger day by day, yet still compact and cozy.

And one day, an energetic burst, and unfolding.

A glorious array of soft, colourful, fragrant petals.

Dancing in the sunlight, fluttering in the gentle breeze. (pause)

Inspired by the light. Dancing in the light.

Become aware of the beauty you share. (long pause)

As you dance in the sun and breeze, notice for a moment that you are firmly rooted in the rich earth you came from.

The rich earth where you will one day return home and begin the beautiful journey again.

This rich soil gives you strength. To begin, to grow, to blossom, to give back.

Its nutrients have become your roots, your stem, your leaves and blossom. The earth and you are one. (pause)

Take a moment in gratitude for the rich earth of your being. (long pause)

Now look above, to the light. The radiant sunshine inspires you. To play, to grow, to blossom, to give back.

Its light has become your roots, your stem, your leaves and blossom.

The sun and you are one. (pause)

Take a moment in gratitude for the radiant sunshine of your being. (long pause)

And now, allow your awareness to rest in its own Self.

Feel the peace in this moment.

Dive deep into the peace, for the next several minutes. (pause 2-10 minutes)

Externalization

And now, preparing to move awareness back out of your floral body. Know that you can return awareness back to this experience again, any time you like. (long pause)

Awareness flies up toward the blue sky.

Look back to see your being as the radiant, strong, beautiful flower.

Leaving your flower body, the experience you had remains in your awareness. Carry any positive feelings or insights with you, into the blue sky, over the vast meadow, back to where your human body is resting. (long pause)

Awareness coming back now, to your human body.

See your body resting peacefully. (pause)

Bring awareness back into the physical body. (pause)

Bringing awareness back into the body.

Bring awareness to the nostrils.

Awareness of the nostrils.

Awareness of the sound of your body breathing. (long pause)

Awareness of any other sounds. (long pause)

Noticing the textures of fabric on your skin. (long pause)

Feel the surface beneath you. (long pause)

Allow awareness to explore the space around you. Sensing the size of the space... the light in the space... the objects nearby... the colours. (pause)

Awareness back in the body, back in the room.

Yoga Nidra is now complete. (pause)

Taking a few deep breaths now and notice sensation coming back to the body. (long pause)

Wiggle your fingers and toes. Feel energy back in the body.

Stretch or move your body any way you like. (long pause)

And if you're lying down, when you're ready, roll to your right side. Take a few deep breaths. (long pause)

Remembering any experiences from your Yoga Nidra practice today. What would you like to take with you? If you don't remember anything, that's fine too. (long pause)

If you were lying down, keeping your eyes closed if you can, press yourself up to sitting. (long pause)

Take a few deep breaths here, feeling awareness back in your body. (long pause)

We'll finish by chanting Om and Shanti three times each.

Feel the energy rise within you as you chant, just as you rose toward the light in your flower body. (pause)

Take a deep breath in.

Om Om Om Shanti Shanti Shanti (pause)

Carry any positive sensations from your Yoga Nidra experience into the rest of your day, open your eyes when you're ready.

Awakening Creativity *(35-55 min.)*

Awaken to the unlimited well of creativity within.

Suggested Pre- and Post-Practices:

- This practice includes time for journaling/sketching, so ask participants to bring supplies for that, or provide them.

- Prepare with a yoga or movement practice that leaves space for creativity and choice. For example, give several variation options for each yoga pose, or try some exploratory/expressive movement –creating waves with various parts of the body, inner exploration of areas of tension and how to release them through movement, or expressing a variety of music through movement.

- Prepare with a progression of bija mantras, moving through the elemental energies from gross to subtle – LAM, VAM, RAM, YAM, HAM, OM. You can include meditation on the chakras from the root (Muladhara) up to the third eye (Ajna), holding silence for awareness of the crown chakra (Sahasrara)

Settling

Getting comfortable for this Yoga Nidra practice to awaken creativity – lying on your back or if it's not comfortable, lying on your side, or sitting up, supported. (pause)

Using any props you need for a soothing set-up. Cushion under your head, blanket to cover you, something under your knees, scarf over your eyes, extra clothing to feel cozy – anything you need. (long pause for settling)

Now checking in – are there any adjustments needed or did you get it just right?

Does your set-up make you feel like you just don't want to leave? Like you're happily melting into relaxation?

If not, what could you do to make it feel more like that? Any adjustments you need are welcome, even if they're different than what I suggested.

Really listen in. What feels right? What's needed? This is *your* practice. To do in your own way. (long pause)

Now that you're settled in, all the effort has ended. There's nothing else you need to do.

If at any time you need to move, then go ahead and do that. Or if it feels restful, enjoy these sweet moments of doing nothing. Getting comfortable for this practice of non-doing. (pause)

Also set aside any notions of "I should" or "I shouldn't". Whatever way you experience this practice is perfect as-is. (pause)

Let go of any struggle with the mind. If it wanders off in a particular way, let it. Simply observe. Watching your experience like watching a bouncy little puppy. With love, laughter, and interest. (pause)

There are no rules to follow. Simply enjoy the journey and notice what happens along the way. (pause)

Beginning a check now that each body part is as relaxed as can be. If you can't completely relax, that's fine. You're welcome just as you are.

Check that your feet and ankles are relaxed as can be. (pause)

Calves, knees and thighs relaxed as can be. (pause)

Hips relaxed as can be. (pause)

Lower back, middle back, upper back releasing tension. Whole back, melting. (pause)

Hands and arms letting go. (pause)

Shoulders and neck melting, tension diffusing. (pause)

Jaw, tongue and cheeks softening. (pause)

Eyes, forehead and scalp softening. (pause)

Whole body melting into the support beneath you. (pause)

Nothing for you to do. (pause)

Notice the sensation of the body resting.

Notice awareness becoming more and more subtle.

Body will sleep, yet awareness continues on.

Effortless awareness.

Awake and aware. (pause)

Now beginning to turn the senses inward.

Become aware of scent in the room. Any scent in the room. (pause)

Light scent, heavy scent, old scent, new scent.

Any scent you are aware of. (long pause)

Maybe scent close to you. The scent of your clothing… your hair… the scent within your nostrils. (long pause)

Moving on to visualization. Visualize the room. The size of the room. (pause)

The shape of the room. (pause) The height of the room. (pause) The colours in the room. (long pause) The shapes in the room. (long pause)

Feel the temperature of the room. Feel the temperature on your hands, feet, cheeks. (long pause) Feel the temperature of the air moving through your nostrils. (long pause)

Be aware of sounds. Be aware of the furthest sounds you can hear. (long pause)

Now be aware of sounds within the room. (long pause)

And finally, be aware of the sound of your own body breathing. (long pause)

Stay effortless.

Effortless awareness.

Simply noticing. (pause)

Yoga Nidra has now begun. (pause)

Rotation of Consciousness

Now awareness moves around the body.

Awareness dancing from place to place.

You can experience this play of awareness in any way you like. (pause)

Move awareness over to the right hand

Right hand thumb

Index finger

Middle finger

Ring finger

Little finger

Moving over to the left hand thumb

Index finger

Middle finger

Ring finger

Little finger

And now over to the right wrist

Left wrist

Right elbow

Left elbow

Right shoulder

Left shoulder

Hollow of the throat

Back of the head near the top

Crown of the head

Eyebrow centre
Right eyebrow
Left eyebrow
Right eye
Left eye
Right ear
Left ear
Right cheek
Left cheek
Tip of the nose
Upper lip
Lower lip
Chin
Hollow of the throat
Heart centre
Right side of the chest
Heart centre
Left side of the chest
Heart centre
Navel centre
Lower abdomen
Right hip
Left hip
Right knee
Left knee
Right ankle
Left ankle
Right big toe
Second toe

Third toe

Fourth toe

Little toe

Left big toe

Second toe

Third toe

Fourth toe

Little toe

The whole right side of the body (pause)

The whole left side of the body (pause)

The whole front of the body (pause)

The whole back of the body (pause)

The whole body together

The whole body together

The whole body together (long pause)

Breath Awareness

Now bring awareness to your spine.

Awareness of the back of your spine.

Bring awareness to your tailbone.

Move awareness inside the tailbone.

Awareness moves from the inside of the tailbone, up through the sacrum, traveling through the centre of the spine, up through the lower spine, middle spine, upper spine to the top of the neck.

Now awareness moves down from the top of the spine, down through the vertebrae of the neck, the upper spine, middle spine, lower spine, through the sacrum to the tip of the tailbone.

Moving through the centre of the spine from the tailbone up to the top of the neck, then from the top of the neck, down to the tip of the tailbone.

Coordinating with each breath.

Each natural breath.

No need to change the breath, simply allow awareness to travel.

Inhale up the spine.

Exhale down the spine.

Experiencing this in any way.

Awareness moving up the spine and down the spine with each breath.

If it feels good, counting the breaths.

Inhale up, 1.

Exhale down, 2.

Inhale up, 3.

Exhale down, 4.

And so on, up to 16. (pause for 1 minute)

Now let go of counting.

It's not important whether you reached 16 or if the mind wandered. There are no expectations.

Now move awareness to the left nostril.

Be aware of inhalation in the left nostril.

Follow inhalation through the left nostril, exhalation through right.

Inhale left

Exhale right

And again, if it feels good, counting the breaths.

Inhale left, 1.

Exhale right, 2.

Inhale left, 3.

Exhale right, 4.

And so on, up to 16. (pause for 1 minute)

Now let go of counting.

It's not important whether you reached 16 or if the mind wandered. There are no expectations.

Letting go of the count. (pause)

Opposites

Now bring awareness to the tip of your nose.

Awareness of the tip of your nose. (pause)

Noticing focused awareness of the tip of your nose.

Focused awareness. (pause)

Now expand awareness to the whole body, all at once.

Expand awareness to the whole body.

Awareness of the whole body. (pause)

Notice diffused awareness.

Diffused awareness. (pause)

Now bring awareness back to the tip of your nose. Notice awareness focusing. (pause)

And allow awareness to expand out to the whole body. Notice awareness diffusing. (pause)

Move back and forth between these two.

Awareness of the tip of the nose, focused.

Awareness of the whole body, diffused.

Awareness of the tip of the nose, tightened.

Awareness of the whole body, open, relaxed. (pause)

Allow awareness to expand out to this open, diffused awareness.

Resting in open, diffused awareness.

Effortless. (long pause)

Symbols

Now expanding into the realm of endless creativity.

Limitless imagination.

Infinite inspiration.

Allowing the vast store of impressions from the subconscious mind to surface.

As symbols are named, images, thoughts, memories or feelings might arise – or maybe nothing will arise.

Either way, simply be the witness. Be effortless.

Not thinking, just watching. (pause)

A bright blue sky (repeat 3 times)

Clear blue waters (repeat 3 times)

Navy blue suit (repeat 3 times)

A closed black umbrella (repeat 3 times)

A yellow umbrella from above (repeat 3 times)

The underside of a green umbrella (repeat 3 times)

A shiny red apple (repeat 3 times)

A shiny red apple rolling (repeat 3 times)

A shiny red apple rolling down a steep hill (repeat 3 times)

Smooth frosting on a cake (repeat 3 times)

Wavy frosting on a cake (repeat 3 times)

Spiky frosting on a cake (repeat 3 times)

A crowded street (repeat 3 times)

And endless ocean (repeat 3 times)

A peaceful valley (repeat 3 times)

If any inspiration, ideas, interesting thoughts arose, take them with you. If not, that's also fine. Know this time has been useful in awakening your creativity and imagination. (pause)

Bring awareness to the point between your eyebrows.

Effortless awareness of the point between the eyebrows.

The third eye.

The eye of intuition.

Continue being the witness. Effortless watching. Sensations might arise, thoughts, ideas, inspiration. Or you might experience it as a peaceful void or unlimited expanse. There is no incorrect way to experience. Simply hold awareness of whatever *is*. Allowing awareness to rest here for the next several minutes. (pause for 5-10 minutes)

Externalization

Ommmmmm

If your mind wandered off, bring awareness back to the point between the eyebrows.

Awareness of the point between the eyebrows. (pause)

Now move awareness down to the nostrils.

Effortless awareness of the nostrils. (pause)

Take a moment to enjoy the effortlessness of your breathing. (pause)

Now take a deep breath.

Feel energy and awareness coming back into the body. (pause)

Yoga Nidra is now complete. (pause)

Take another deep breath. (pause)

Begin moving your body. Small movements, then larger movements. Bringing awareness fully into the body now.

Moving however you'd like. Awakening back into the body, however you'd like. (pause)

And if you like, take a moment to recall your experience. Seeds of inspiration and ideas were planted. Are there any you're aware of, or that stand out in your mind? (long pause)

Making a choice now – for the next several minutes, either continue resting, maybe in a different position if you like, or open your eyes, and write down or sketch any thoughts, ideas or curiosities that you don't want to forget. Making your choice when you're ready. (pause for 3-10 minutes)

And now, wrapping up your rest, your writing or sketching. Prepare to return to sitting upright. (pause for 30 seconds)

Return to sitting upright now, taking a moment to enjoy any positive experience from your Yoga Nidra practice today. (long pause)

Thanking yourself for practicing and diving into the unlimited well of creativity. (pause)

I'll finish by chanting Om and Shanti three times each. Join in if you like.

Notice your energy rising with the chant.

Take a deep breath in.

Om Om Om Shanti Shanti Shanti (pause)

Take a moment to appreciate all of the sensory awareness coming back to you – sounds, textures, scent. Being aware of the senses reactivated. When you're ready, open your eyes. Have an inspired day.

Free Gift!

Here's an opportunity to enjoy three of my Yoga Nidra mp3 recordings, for free.

3 Free Audio Recordings

Let me lull you into sweet relaxation, rejuvenation and reconnection with some of my most popular Yoga Nidra practices:

- Anytime Calming
- Overflowing Heart Yoga Nidra
- Rainbow Light Yoga Nidra

Get them at tamaraskyhawk.com/free now!

Reviews Appreciated!

Enjoy the book?
Sharing a review on Amazon is incredibly helpful in spreading the goodness. Help more people learn about the book and benefit.

Leave your review on Amazon now!

With much gratitude,
Tamara

Printed in Great Britain
by Amazon